Complications in Ophthalmic Plastic Surgery

Springer Science+Business Media, LLC

Brian G. Brazzo, MD

Clinical Assistant Professor of Ophthalmology, Weill Medical College of Cornell University, New York, New York

Editor

Complications in Ophthalmic Plastic Surgery

With 117 Illustrations in 141 Parts, 116 in Full Color

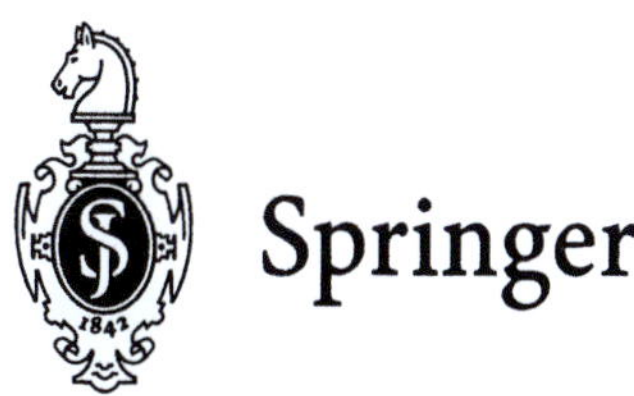

Springer

Brian G. Brazzo, MD
Clinical Assistant Professor of Ophthalmology
Weill Medical College of Cornell University
New York, NY 10021
USA

Library of Congress Cataloging-in-Publication Data
Complications in ophthalmic plastic surgery / editor, Brian G. Brazzo.
   p. ; cm.
   Includes bibliographical references and index.
   ISBN 978-1-4419-1813-0   ISBN 978-0-387-21654-6 (eBook)
   DOI 10.1007/978-0-387-21654-6
   1. Ophthalmic plastic surgery—Complications. I. Brazzo, Brian G.
   [DNLM: 1. Ophthalmologic Surgical Procedures—adverse effects. 2. Surgery,
Plastic—adverse effects. WW 168 C7368 2003]
   RE87.C665 2003
   617.7′1—dc21   2002044510

Printed on acid-free paper

9 8 7 6 5 4 3 2 1   SPIN 10905241

www.springer-ny.com

Foreword

Since 1985, it has been my privilege to be the Director of The Society of Byron Smith Fellows. During the years in which Byron Smith was with us, his former fellows would meet at the American Academy of Ophthalmology's annual meeting. They would present to him, and to one another, interesting cases of their own complications that had occurred or cases that had been sent to them that were complications to be repaired. This forum provided the fellows with an excellent format for evaluating their own problems and also for discussing how to treat extremely difficult cases.

Shortly after Dr. Brian Brazzo completed his fellowship with me in 1998, he asked if I thought it would be appropriate for him to edit a new book on complications of ophthalmic plastic surgery. Certainly, during his fellowship, it became apparent that Dr. Brazzo was probably the most gifted academician and writer that I had ever had the pleasure of training and meeting. I could think of no one more appropriate to continue the work initiated by Dr. Byron Smith and carried on by his students.

I believe that the group of authors Dr. Brazzo has assembled to produce this book are among the finest oculoplastic surgeons that have ever been trained. There can be no doubt that this is a wonderful adjunct to the oculoplastic literature and fills a void in the current literature by providing a comprehensive text on the treatment of complications in ophthalmic plastic surgery.

Frank A. Nesi, MD, FAACS

PREFACE

Complications are an unavoidable reality of surgery. Even with meticulous evaluation, preparation, and technique, unforeseen events do occur. When events do not proceed as planned, perhaps experience is the best guide to overcoming obstacles. Certainly, a thorough knowledge of surgical technique and an ability to appropriately discuss the circumstances with the patient are also important in achieving a satisfactory outcome.

Complications mean different things to different people. Some surgeons seem unconcerned with events other than the life-threatening or vision-impairing variety. Other surgeons, and patients, may be concerned with mild asymmetry or subtle irregularities that would not be perceived by a casual observer.

Even surgeons disagree on what constitutes an acceptable outcome. I have seen speakers at conferences present pre- and postoperative pictures. Frequently, blepharoplasty produces dramatic changes, but underlying ptosis is often ignored or made worse. While some surgeons are impressed with the outcome following skin removal, eye plastic surgeons might consider such results unacceptable and in need of revision.

There are many excellent books that detail the surgical procedures covered in this book. Most, however, give only brief reference to complications and their management. This text covers evaluation and management of complications associated with the most common reconstructive and aesthetic procedures in ophthalmic plastic surgery.

The chapters all have a similar outline, with sections for evaluation, technique, and complications. The evaluation and technique sections cover the necessary steps for their respective procedures but provide special attention to preventing complications. The complications section is intended to exemplify the most appropriate medical and surgical management for postoperative patients. Throughout the text, potential difficulties are identified and followed by discussion on prevention and treatment.

The contributing authors have provided their expertise in dealing with the topics. Our goals are to communicate the most common and significant complications associated with surgery, and to instruct surgeons how to prevent and deal with unforeseen events. We have selected topics that residents and fellows in facial surgery, ophthalmologists, and other surgical specialists will commonly encounter. We hope that these recommendations will improve surgical outcomes, and perhaps be a substitute for adversity.

Brian G. Brazzo, MD

ACKNOWLEDGMENTS

I appreciate the help that the contributors provided and am grateful for their insight and participation. Laurel Craven, Executive Editor, provided motivation, suggestions, and direction from the earliest stages of planning. Christine Park, Assistant Editor, has done an excellent job in organizing and coordinating activities among the authors and various departments. I am thankful for the assistance of the entire staff at Springer-Verlag, especially the production department, which has helped to reformat the numerous images and give this book its current appearance. I also appreciate the help of Chernow Editorial Services, which helped to place the final touches on the manuscript.

Finally, I will always be thankful for the examples which my preceptors, Frank A. Nesi, MD, and Geoffrey J. Gladstone, MD, set during my years of fellowship. In thousands of procedures with them, they always achieved the best possible outcome. Their dedication to ophthalmic and facial plastic surgery and their commitment to excellence have been motivating me throughout my career.

Brian G. Brazzo, MD

CONTENTS

Part I   Cosmetic Surgery

Part II   Ptosis

Part III Lower Eyelid Malposition

                                                            Contents

CONTRIBUTORS

Richard L. Anderson, MD
Medical Director, Center for Facial Appearances, Salt Lake City, UT 84102, USA

Brian G. Brazzo, MD
Clinical Assistant Professor of Ophthalmology, Weill Medical College of Cornell University, New York, NY 10021; and Director, Oculoplastics Service, Department of Ophthalmology, Maimonides Medical Center, Brooklyn, NY 11219, USA

Daniel E. Buerger, MD
Clinical Instructor of Ophthalmology, University of Pittsburgh School of Medicine, Pittsburgh, PA 15213, USA

Steven Chen, MD
Clinical Assistant Professor, Department of Ophthalmology, Tulane University School of Medicine, New Orleans, LA 70112; and Clinical Lecturer, Department of Ophthalmology, University of Arizona Health Sciences Center, Tucson, AZ 85724, USA

Adam J. Cohen, MD
Consulting Surgeon, St. Vincent Hospital, Santa Fe, NM 87505, USA

Briggs E. Cook, Jr., MD
Charlotte Ophthalmology Center for Sight, Charlotte, NC 28211, USA

Kip Dolphin, MD
Assistant Professor of Ophthalmology, Weill Medical College of Cornell University, New York, NY 10021, USA

Geoffrey J. Gladstone, MD, FAACS
Clinical Professor of Ophthalmology, Michigan State University School of
Medicine, East Lansing, MI 48824; Assistant Clinical Professor of
Ophthalmology and Otolaryngology, Kesge Eye Institute, Wayne State
University School of Medicine, Detroit, MI 48201; Co-Director,
Oculoplastic Surgery, Department of Ophthalmology, William Beaumont
Hospital, Royal Oak, MI 48073; and Consultants in Ophthalmic and
Facial Plastic Surgery, Southfield, MI 48034, USA

Jemshed A. Khan, MD
Clinical Professor of Ophthalmology, Kansas University School of Medicine,
Kansas City, KS 66160; and Director, Khan Eyelid and Facial Plastic
Surgery, Overland Park, KS 64111, USA

Taj G. Khan, DO
Ophthalmic Plastic and Reconstructive Surgery, Associated Eye Physicians
and Surgeons of New Jersey, Union, NJ 07950, USA

Jessica Lattman, MD
Department of Ophthalmology, Manhattan Eye, Ear & Throat Hospital,
New York, NY 10021, USA

Bradley N. Lemke, MD, FACS
Clinical Professor, Department of Ophthalmology and Visual Sciences,
University of Wisconsin School of Medicine, Madison, WI 53792; and
Lemke Facial Surgery, Madison, WI 53717, USA

Mark J. Lucarelli, MD
Assistant Clinical Professor, Oculoplastics Service, Department of
Ophthalmology and Visual Sciences, University of Wisconsin School of
Medicine, Madison, WI 53792, USA

Michael Mercandetti, MD, MBA, FACS
Midtown Medical Plaza, Sarasota, FL 34241, USA

Frank A. Nesi, MD, FAACS
Director, Oculoplastic Surgery, Beaumont Eye Institute, Department of
Ophthalmology, William Beaumont Hospital, Royal Oak, MI 48073; and
Consultants in Ophthalmic and Facial Plastic Surgery, Southfield, MI
48034, USA

Cassandra B. Onofrey, MD
Bascom Palmer Eye Institute, University of Miami School of Medicine,
Miami, FL 33136, USA

Julian D. Perry, MD
Associate Staff, Division of Ophthalmology, Cole Eye Institute Departments
of Ophthalmic Plastic and Orbital Surgery and Neuro-Ophthalmology,
The Cleveland Clinic Foundation, Cleveland, OH 44195, USA

David Rosenberg, MD
Department of Otolaryngology and Facial Plastic Surgery, Manhattan Eye,
Ear & Throat Hospital, New York, NY 10021, USA

Norman Shorr, MD, FACS
Clinical Professor of Ophthalmology; Director, Fellowship on Ophthalmic
and Orbital Plastic and Reconstructive Surgery; and Director, Aesthetic
Reconstructive Surgery Service, Jules Stein Eye Institute, University of
California, Los Angeles, CA 90210, USA

César A. Sierra, MD
Department of Ophthalmology, Yale University School of Medicine, New
Haven, CT 06520, USA

Richard A. Stangler, MD
Director, Ophthalmic Plastic and Reconstructive Service, Fox Eye Laser
and Cosmetic Institute; and Chairman, Ophthalmology Department,
St. Luke's Hospital, Cedar Rapids, IA 52406, USA

George O. Stasior, MD, FACS
Clinical Professor, Division of Eye Plastic & Reconstructive Surgery,
Department of Ophthalmology, Albany Medical College, Albany,
NY 12110, USA

Orkan George Stasior, MD, FACS
Clinical Professor, Division of Eye Plastic & Reconstructive Surgery,
Department of Ophthalmology, Albany Medical College, Albany,
NY 12110, USA

David T. Tse, MD, FACS
Professor, Department of Ophthalmology, Bascom Palmer Eye Institute,
University of Miami School of Medicine, Miami, FL 33136, USA

Michael T. Yen, MD
Assistant Professor of Ophthalmology, Cullen Eye Institute, Baylor College
of Medicine, Houston, TX 77030, USA

PART I

COSMETIC SURGERY

UPPER BLEPHAROPLASTY

• Jemshed A. Khan

Dermatochalasis, or excess upper eyelid skin, is a very common condition that progresses with age. Upper blepharoplasty, which removes this excess tissue and modifies the contour of the lid, may be indicated on the basis of functional impairment, cosmetic concerns, or both. Cosmetic blepharoplasty is among the most common aesthetic surgical procedures in this country and may be performed as an isolated surgery or in conjunction with other eyelid and facial procedures.

EVALUATION

Evaluation of the upper blepharoplasty candidate begins with the history, which probes for the patient's desired surgical outcome and tolerance for imperfection. Most patients desire a reduction of bulging fat pads, an exposed band of pretarsal skin, and absence of lateral hooding. The surgeon should demonstrate with a mirror what can be accomplished with surgery.

The surgeon should inquire about risk factors that could compromise the surgical result. Standard presurgical questions examine the use of drugs such as aspirin, Coumadin, nonsteroidal anti-inflammatory drugs (NSAIDs), or antiplatelet drugs that may increase the risk of intraoperative or postoperative bleeding. Such drugs are often discontinued for an appropriate interval prior to elective surgery. Patients at a higher risk for postoperative corneal epithelial keratopathy include those with dry eye symptoms, facial nerve palsy (including Bell's palsy), and prior blepharoplasty.

The examination begins with measurements of the margin reflex distance (MRD1, the distance, in millimeters, from the central corneal light reflex to the upper eyelid margin) with and without the eyebrows manually raised. This test will uncover any underlying true eyelid ptosis. The surgeon should inform the patient that the MRD1 obtained with eyebrows manually raised is highly predictive of the postblepharoplasty MRD1.[1]

While the brows are manually raised, the superior sulcus is examined for evidence of herniating nasal and preaponeurotic fat pads, and of prolapsed lacrimal gland. Balloting the globe while examining the superior sulcus may help determine which fat pads should be resected. Any preexisting eyebrow ptosis, eyelid ptosis, or nasal webbing should be documented and emphasized to the patient. Finally, the extent of lateral hooding and retro–orbicularis oculi fat (ROOF) should be noted.

The surgeon should determine if lagophthalmos is present by having the patient passively close the eyelids as if sleeping. At the same time, the Bell's phenomenon should be examined. With the eyelids gently closed, the examiner gently opens the lids and inspects the position of the globe. A superior rotation of the globe ("positive Bell's") indicates better corneal protection during sleep and blinking. Slit lamp corneal evaluation with rose bengal or fluorescein epithelial staining, as well as Schirmer's tear test, helps screen for dry eye.

Following this examination, the surgeon should have a clear understanding of the patient's expectations, surgical risk factors, and underlying anatomical eyelid changes. With this information, the surgeon may negotiate a surgical plan that safely meets the patient's needs and expectations.

TECHNIQUE

Upper blepharoplasty requires an incisional device such as a scalpel, scissors, carbon dioxide (CO_2) laser, electrosurgery tip, or radiofrequency tip. Other useful instruments include a millimeter ruler, 0.3 mm toothed forceps, needle holder, hemostat, and cautery. Depending on the incisional method, special protective devices such as nonconductive or metal globe shields and guards may be needed.

When marking the eyelid skin for excision, the surgeon must always remember that the inferior border of the skin incision usually becomes the postoperative eyelid crease. If the inferior incisions are misplaced or asymmetrical, the final results will reflect these errors. Therefore, careful skin markings are critical. In Caucasian eyelids, the inferior incision is usually marked in the preexisting crease, which is normally 9 to 11 mm superior to the central eyelid margin, 4 mm superior to the upper punctum, and 6 mm superior to the lateral canthal angle. These markings may be lower in Asian eyelids (see Chapter 5). The female eyelid usually has a crease that is higher than that of the male eyelid and demonstrates a greater arch. The eyelid crease (and inferior marking) usually curves somewhat downward as it extends toward the medial and lateral canthi (Fig. 1.1).

With the patient supine, the surgeon uses the "pinch" technique to determine the amount of skin removal. Excess skin is gently

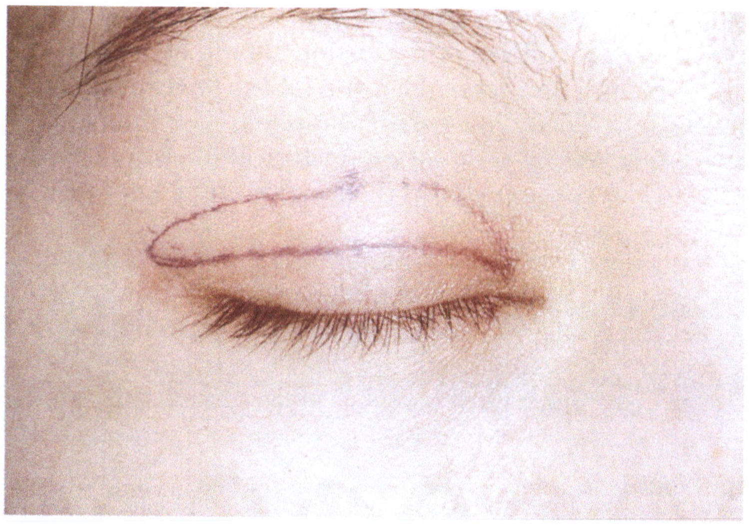

FIGURE 1.1. Preblepharoplasty skin marking on right upper eyelid. The inferior resection margin is the anticipated new eyelid crease. The medial extent of removal is superior to the punctum. The lateral extent is often determined by degree of hooding and may be limited by the lateral orbital rim. (Reproduced with permission from Khan JA. Laser Blepharoplasty. In: Chen WP, ed. *Oculoplastic Surgery: The Essentials.* New York: Thieme; 2001:15–77.)

grasped with forceps and the eyelid position is noted. The surgeon confirms that the lids can passively close. The inferior aspect of the skin flap generally corresponds to the lid crease. The medial extent of the incision is often superior to the punctum but should be moved laterally if there is a tendency for medial canthal webbing. The lateral extent of removal is often determined by hooding and may be limited by the lateral orbital rim.

Perhaps the most important aspect of the marking involves leaving an appropriate amount of tissue to prevent lagophthalmos. The surgeon will seldom encounter significant problems in the postoperative phase if adequate skin remains at the conclusion of the case. Generally, at least 1 cm of skin should remain inferior to the inferior incision, and at least 1 cm should be left between the superior marking and the brow. If less than 2 cm of tissue remains between the brow and lid margin, there will be a higher possibility of lagophthalmos. Also, there will be a greater chance of aesthetic irregularity if the thin eyelid skin is sutured to the darker, thicker sub-brow skin. If skin excision under these parameters does not appear to create the desired eyelid appearance, then the surgeon should consider other options, such as browlift (see Chapter 4).

The upper aspect of the skin excision should be a gentle arch that connects the medial and lateral borders of the lower incision. This upper border can be easily lowered if the pinch test indicates that eyelid closure might not be adequate following skin closure. The surgeon should then mark the margins of the flap and remeasure with calipers to ensure symmetry.

Local anesthesia with or without intravenous sedation provides adequate patient comfort for blepharoplasty. Sublingual diazepam (5.0 mg tab) helps reduce anxiety when the procedure is performed entirely under local anesthesia. Typical local anesthetic consists of 2% lidocaine with epinephrine (1:200,000), mixed with an equal volume of 0.75% bupivicaine hydrochloride (Marcaine). For better diffusion, hyaluronidase (Wydase) is often added to the infiltrate. After 10 to 20 minutes, the epinephrine provides improved hemostasis.

When incising the skin and orbicularis, the surgeon should be aware of the position of the levator aponeurosis, which may be directly beneath the orbicularis at the inferior incision. The author usually excises skin and orbicularis as a single specimen, but separate layered excision is acceptable. When one excises the skin–muscle ellipse, light traction and countertraction should be applied while the surgical plane is sharply developed with Westcott scissors or other incisional device.

The dissection plane must remain at the level of the postorbicularis fascia. If the incision is carried deeper, the levator can easily be transected. The surgeon should always inspect the deeper tissue planes after skin and orbicularis excision. If the levator appears to have been transected or disinserted from the tarsus, it should be repaired with one or two simple interrupted sutures.

Next, if fat excision is planned, the orbital septum is opened laterally by creating a "buttonhole" in the septum through which fat prolapses freely (Fig. 1.2). It is often helpful to apply light pressure to the globe to better inspect and visualize the underlying (preaponeurotic) postseptal fat pockets. The entire horizontal width of the exposed septum may be divided.

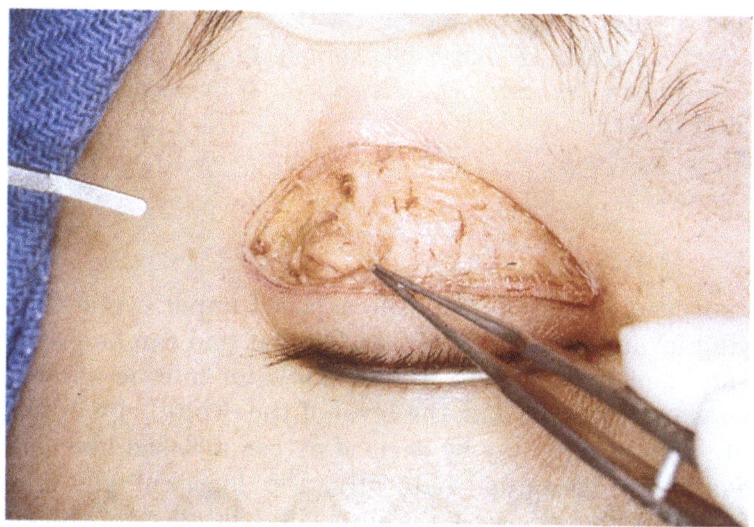

FIGURE 1.2. The orbital septum should be incised along its entire horizontal width. To confirm the location of the septum, the surgeon can grasp the septum with forceps and gently pull inferiorly. A firm attachment to the orbital rim, as demonstrated, confirms identification of the septum. (Reproduced with permission from Khan JA. Laser blepharoplasty. In: Chen WP, ed. *Oculoplastic Surgery: The Essentials*. New York: Thieme; 2001:15–77.)

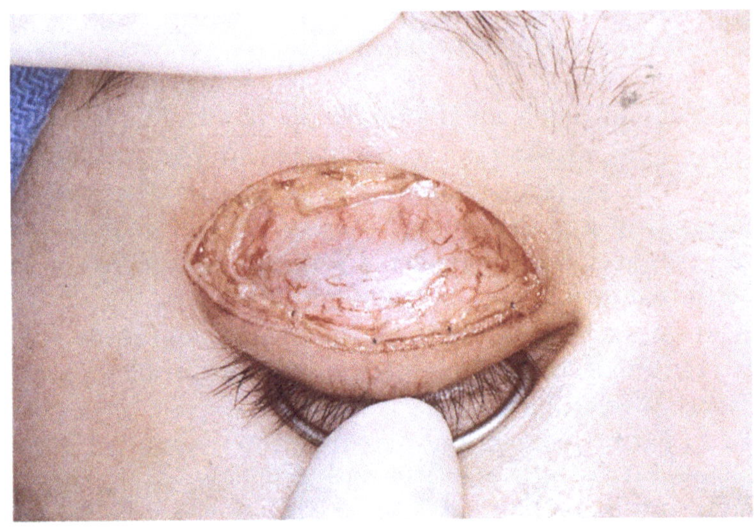

FIGURE 1.3. The fat pads are located posterior to the septum and superior to the levator muscle. (Reproduced with permission from Khan JA. Laser blepharoplasty. In: Chen WP, ed. *Oculoplastic Surgery: The Essentials.* New York: Thieme; 2001:15–77.)

The surgeon should identify the exposed upper eyelid fat pad and underlying levator muscle (Fig. 1.3). The fat pad can be grasped with forceps and gently separated from the levator muscle and aponeurosis. The fat pad is excised at the level of the orbital rim or Whitnall's ligament. The fat pad may be excised across a closed hemostat or divided against a backstop. Laterally, the lacrimal gland must be avoided. Adequate hemostasis is important because of the caliber of vessels associated with the fat pocket (Fig. 1.4).

Next, the nasal fat pad is approached by bluntly spreading the fascia over the nasal fat pad with a hemostat. Balloting the globe will often bring the fat pad forward. If the fat is not adequately exposed, the surgeon can make an X-shaped incision over the nasal fat pad and deepen the incision until fat prolapses. The protruding fat can be bluntly separated from surrounding tissue with a cotton-tipped applicator. The base of the nasal fat pad usually requires supplemental local anesthesia injection prior to excision. The fat pad may be ex-

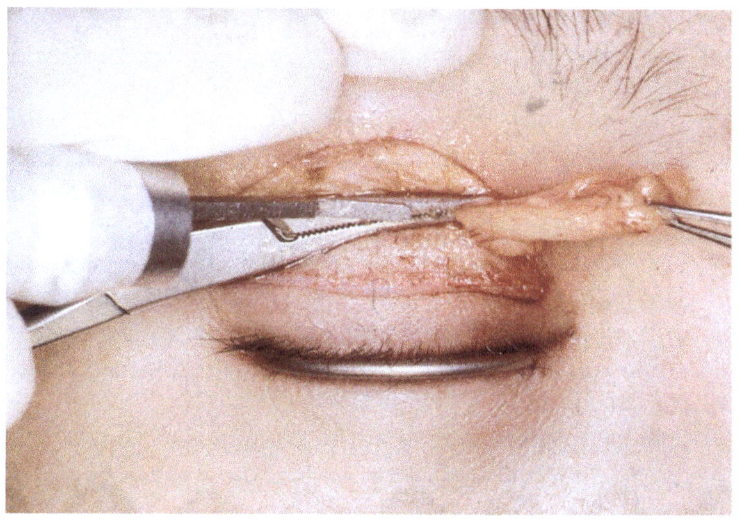

FIGURE 1.4. Preaponeurotic fat is excised. (Reproduced with permission from Khan JA. Laser blepharoplasty. In: Chen WP, ed. *Oculoplastic Surgery: The Essentials*. New York: Thieme; 2001:15–77.)

cised across a closed hemostat, or divided against a backstop. Again, the surgeon must ensure adequate hemostasis.

If a small amount of protruding orbital fat is present, it may be reduced by applying cautery directly to the fat pad. The surgeon can visualize the retraction of the tissue. When skin–orbicularis excision is emphasized, cautery reduction of fat may be accomplished without opening the orbital septum. Cautery applied to the tissue covering the fat will accomplish the same result.

If necessary, the ROOF fat may be excised. The surgeon should grasp the upper wound edge and gently pull inferiorly. Sharp scissors dissection is carried superiorly, toward the brow, in the suborbicularis plane. At the level of the superior orbital rim, ROOF can be visualized when the skin flap is elevated. The ROOF can be excised from the deep connective tissue overlying the orbital rim. Bare periosteum should not be exposed, to prevent adhesion to the skin. Cautery is applied to any bleeding vessels.

One method of skin closure involves interrupted 6-0 polypropylene (Prolene) suture nasally and running 6-0 Prolene for remainder (Fig. 1.5), with attention to take only superficial dermal bites (0.5 mm depth) to reduce bleeding. Some surgeons attempt to recreate the eyelid crease by placing three interrupted sutures that incorporate dermis and orbicularis of the upper skin edge, and the surface of the levator aponeurosis along the superior tarsal border. Deeper (1.5 mm depth) bites are taken lateral to the canthal angle to reduce the risk of wound dehiscence. Use of a tapered needle may reduce bleeding. Ointment is applied to the incision and to the inferior cul-de-sac if the patient has not regained full eyelid closure. Sutures can be removed after 7 to 15 days.

Postoperative instructions include application of ice compresses frequently, erythromycin ointment to the incision once per day, and avoidance of strenuous activity.

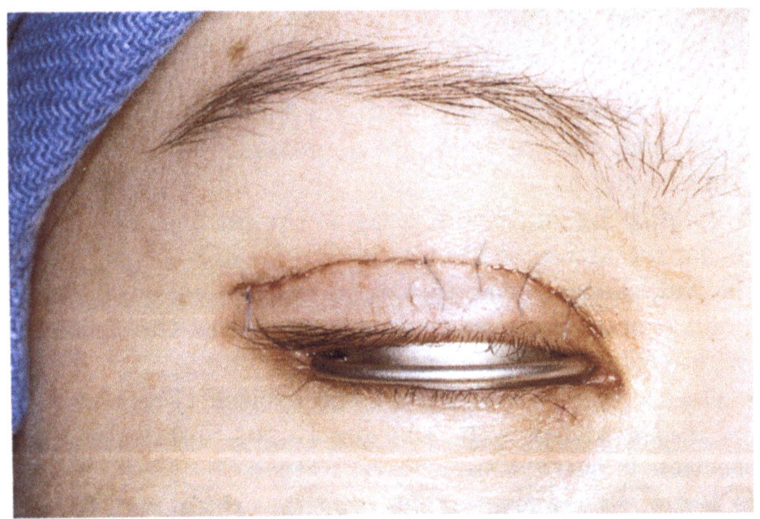

FIGURE 1.5. The skin incision is closed with interrupted 6-0 Prolene suture nasally and running 6-0 Prolene for the remainder, with attention to take only superficial dermal bites to reduce bleeding. (Reproduced with permission from Khan JA. Laser blepharoplasty. In: Chen WP, ed. *Oculoplastic Surgery: The Essentials*. New York: Thieme; 2001:15–77.)

                                                    Upper Blepharoplasty

COMPLICATIONS

Lagophthalmos following blepharoplasty may reflect a preexisting condition or may be related to surgery. Reassurance alone is appropriate if the lagophthalmos is asymptomatic and corneal epithelial exposure changes are mild. When a patient is symptomatic during the night or upon awakening, the surgeon should suspect nocturnal lagophthalmos, which can be treated with topical lubricant ointment, humidified room air, avoidance of a breeze from fans or ventilation ducts, and taping or patching the eyelids closed at night. When a patient is symptomatic later in the day or in the evening, the surgeon should suspect incomplete or delayed blink. Treatments include artificial tears, punctal plugs, bandage contact lens, and humidified room air.

Beginning about 3 weeks after surgery, all lagophthalmos patients may begin downward massage of the pretarsal upper eyelid to stretch and loosen the tight upper eyelid. Five minutes of downward stretching of the eyelid per waking hour for 12 weeks is prescribed. Stretching may be accomplished with a finger, by the rolling action of a cotton-tipped applicator on the pretarsal skin, or by gently pulling the eyelashes inferiorly.

Additional surgery may be indicated for patients who do not respond to medical management with punctal plugs, develop corneal complications, or have not improved significantly after 3 months. The first step in evaluating such patients is to determine the cause of the lagophthalmos. If the lagophthalmos resolves when the eyebrows as manually pushed inferiorly, the surgeon should suspect a vertical skin deficiency. If the lagophthalmos does not improve while the eyebrows are manually pushed inferiorly, the surgeon should suspect internal adhesions. By pulling inferiorly on the eyelashes, the examiner can determine whether there is a fixed adhesive band. Often, the stress lines caused by taut adhesive bands can be palpated and visualized. When there is eyelid retraction in primary gaze, the cause is usually either excessive levator aponeurosis advancement or internal adhesion to the orbital septum. Rarely, a patient develops a paralytic lagophthalmos.

Vertical skin shortage is treated by placement of a free skin graft. Internal adhesions are treated by exploration, lysis, and excision of adhesions with postoperative Frost suture placement. While significant improvement in blink usually occurs, complete elimination of lagophthalmos or return of normal involuntary blink is unlikely.

Mild ptosis following uncomplicated blepharoplasty may be related to edema or stretching of the levator and often improves spontaneously over 6 to 12 weeks. One should consider surgical ptosis repair if the ptosis persists, is not improving by 6 to 8 weeks after surgery, or if the levator was extremely thin or divided during surgery. Otherwise, as long as there is continuing improvement, patient and surgeon may wait up to 6 months. If the levator is transected intraoperatively, it can be repaired by placing one or two interrupted sutures between the severed ends of the levator, or between the levator and tarsus.

Asymmetric or uneven folds after blepharoplasty may be the result of unequal skin excision, preexisting asymmetry, or an unpredictable drop in the compensatory preoperative position of one or both eyebrows. In straightforward cases, the surgeon can excise additional skin on the side with the lower fold to achieve symmetry. In general, the surgeon excises a vertical height of skin that is twice the amount of asymmetry between the folds. For example, if the right skin fold hangs 2 mm lower than the left, the surgeon should excise a 4 mm vertical skin ellipse from the right eyelid.

When the eyelid creases are asymmetric, one must reset them to a symmetrical height, utilizing lid crease fixation sutures. It is very difficult to lower an eyelid crease, however, and asymmetry is usually addressed by elevating to lower crease. During the reoperation, the crease is drawn at the desired height. Excess skin should be excised above this marking. Several simple interrupted sutures can be placed to appose the skin edges, with incorporation of deeper tissue (levator or tarsus) to accentuate the crease position.

Lateral hooding often recurs despite apparently adequate intraoperative tissue resection. This hooding, probably a result of the eyebrows dropping postoperatively, may be treated by further lateral skin and orbicularis excision. Brow repair (see Chapter 4) should also be considered and may provide a more definitive improvement.

Medial canthal webbing is difficult to correct and often improves gradually over time. Prior to surgery, the "stress test" helps to unmask any tendency for nasal webbing. Manual inferior traction is placed on the mobile skin of the bridge and side of the nose while the medial canthal area is observed for skin movement or web formation. If skin movement or web formation is observed, the medial aspect of the proposed incision is moved lateral to the area of webbing or movement. When webbing persists postoperatively, it may sometimes be repaired with refixation of a weak or descended nasal lid crease with full-thickness 4-0 chromic mattress stitches. Other options include V- to Y-plasty or other epicanthal fold techniques.

The surgeon should always try to prevent medial webbing by being particularly conservative with skin excision. At the end, more skin may be removed if large excess is apparent. During closure, several simple interrupted sutures can be used to close the medial wound. If tension or webbing becomes apparent, the suture(s) should be removed and repositioned so that the skin has appropriate contour without tension. When the medial skin appears in the proper position, a running suture may be used to close the remainder of the wound.

Direct injury to the globe is one of the most dreaded complications of blepharoplasty surgery. The risk of such injuries may be reduced by placement of a shield between the eyelids and globe. However, even when such precautions are employed, the device may become dislodged during surgery, thereafter failing to provide adequate protection. It is not always possible to judge the exact location of the underlying shield during eyelid surgery, and injury may occur when deep dissection is performed beyond the edge of the protective device. This is especially concerning when one is working superior to the insertion of the septum onto the levator aponeurosis.

If globe perforation occurs, the eye must be protected from undue pressure, which might result in expulsion of ocular contents. The patient should be referred immediately for intraocular evaluation. If severe corneal injury occurs, a corneal specialist should be consulted.

Wound dehiscence usually occurs to the segment of the incision lateral to the lateral canthal angle because this area not only supports the weight of the cheek but also is stressed when the face is rubbed against the pillow during sleep. Therefore, the suture bites in this area are 2 mm wide and deep, and include skin and orbicularis. With this technique, the author usually removes skin stitches between the 9th and 14th postoperative days.

When the eyelid skin is closed following upper blepharoplasty, a modified wound closure technique will help to reduce the incidence of dehiscence and bleeding. The author recommends the use of a tapered rather than a cutting needle for suturing, nonabsorbing (i.e., 6-0 Prolene) suture, which will retain its tensile strength, and 0.5 mm bites of skin only (avoiding orbicularis) in the non-tension-bearing portion of the incision that is medial to the lateral canthal angle. Fast-absorbing 6-0 collagen or chromic suture is also quite popular because the dissolving material need not be removed. However, this suture has insufficient tensile strength to permit its use for cutaneous eyelid incisions created by CO_2 laser, radiofrequency, or electrosurgery.

Upper eyelid or retrobulbar hematomas may occur postoperatively despite adequate intraoperative hemostasis. In the author's opinion, such bleeding usually emanates from vessels larger than 0.25 mm that are located on the undersurface of the upper aspect of the wound, often close to the eyebrow or in the nasal aspect. Whenever such vessels are encountered, the author makes a special effort to cauterize them by using bipolar cautery. Large or vision-threatening hematomas will require drainage and are followed by prolonged swelling.

Hematoma with elevated intraocular pressure that threatens perfusion of the central retinal artery is a true ophthalmic emergency that may progress to central artery occlusion and permanent blindness. The surgeon should immediately lower intraocular pressure or reduce orbital pressure. Treatments may include lateral canthotomy and inferior cantholysis, globe massage, orbital exploration and evacuation of hematoma, bony orbital decompression, administration of intravenous and topical drugs to lower intraocular pressure, and anterior chamber paracentesis.[2]

A theoretical risk of blepharoplasty is wound infection. However, in the author's experience, infection is very uncommon and prophylactic oral antibiotics are unnecessary. Following routine cases, topical erythromycin ophthalmic ointment is applied to the incision once daily until sutures are removed.

Even among patients who are prone to keloid formation, hypertrophic scarring is unusual in the thin eyelid skin. The risk of hypertrophic or noticeable scarring may be reduced by avoiding incision placement into adjacent thicker skin and in areas where webbing may occur, and by layering wound closure when wound tension appears unusually high.

Early or delayed scarring is an unusual complication that may be attributed to an exuberant healing response. Very mild scarring may be treated with topical steroids or intralesional triamcinolone (Kenalog) at a concentration of 5 mg/mL (the higher potency ophthalmic preparation may induce dermal atrophy). Application of a silicone gel or sheeting, alone or in combination, or Cordoran tape, may also be helpful. When hypertrophic scarring is minimal to moderate and still vascular, it may respond to 585 nm pulsed dye laser treatment. True keloid formation may respond to intralesional steroids plus 585 nm pulsed dye laser irradiation. Persistent hypertrophic incisional scars may be excised after waiting for 6 months.

REFERENCES

1. Khan JA, Garden V. Blepharoplasty or ptosis repair? Modified preoperative MRD1b measurement predicts post-blepharoplasty MRD1 [abstract]. Proceedings of the 31st Annual Scientific Symposium of the American Society of Ophthalmic Plastic and Reconstructive Surgery. Fall 2000, Dallas, TX.

2. Khan JA. Blunt trauma to orbital soft tissues. In: Shingleton BJ, Hersh P, Kenyon K, eds. *Eye Trauma*. St Louis: Mosby-Year Book; 1991:287–294.

2

LOWER BLEPHAROPLASTY

• Julian D. Perry
• Norman Shorr

The appearance of the lower eyelids is affected by the complex interaction of structures comprising the eyelid, orbit, and midface. The surgeon should consider the lower eyelid to be a continuum that begins at the lid margin and extends to the upper lip. Understanding the dynamic forces that govern lower eyelid position and contour requires a thorough knowledge of lower eyelid, cheek, and nasolabial anatomy.

EVALUATION

Evaluation for lower blepharoplasty begins with a discussion of the patient's desires and technical realities. Surgeon and patient must first determine the desired and possible aesthetic results, then decide which techniques may best achieve those results.

Although lower blepharoplasty may reduce areas of fat bulging superior to the orbital rim, it does not address the area of tissue paucity over the rim or the malar bags. The underlying bony structure may contribute to a concavity inferior to the orbital rim. This bony groove typically extends from the anterior lacrimal crest toward the infraorbital foramen, and it has been termed the "tear trough" abnormality. The tear trough abnormality may exaggerate the double convexity deformity.

Evaluation should include assessment of the underlying bone and sub–orbicularis oculi fat (SOOF) tissues, not just fat and skin. The area of tissue paucity may be treated with concomitant fat repositioning, and the tear trough abnormality may be treated with implant material to fill the bony defect. SOOF and orbicularis ptosis may also be addressed through midface elevation techniques. The choice of procedures to be performed should be made preoperatively. The surgeon assesses the amount of deformity in each layer of the lower eyelid–midface continuum, including skin, muscle, SOOF, orbital fat, and bone. The degree of deformity in each individual layer will determine the optimal combination of procedures to create the desired change.

Preoperative evaluation should include assessment of lower lid tone. Patients with horizontal eyelid laxity are at higher risk for post-blepharoplasty lower eyelid retraction. The distraction and "snapback" tests are useful in the preoperative identification of patients with lower eyelid laxity.

The distraction test is performed by grasping the lower eyelid and pulling it away from the globe. If the lower eyelid can be pulled more than 7 mm from the globe, the distraction test is positive, and horizontal laxity exists. The "snapback" test is performed by pulling the skin of the lower eyelid inferiorly, as shown in Chapter 10 (see Fig. 10.1). If the eyelid does not spontaneously return to its normal anatomical position before the next blink, the snap test is positive, which signifies that the eyelid has diminished tone. The degree of horizontal lower eyelid laxity determines the method of repair.

If minimal horizontal laxity is present and transcutaneous blepharoplasty is performed, lateral canthal tendon tightening (see later: Figs. 2.6 and 10.6) will decrease the chance of significant postoperative eyelid retraction. Moderate to severe horizontal lid laxity should be addressed through lateral canthal resuspension. Finally, the surgeon should understand that removal of redundant skin does not address skin quality. Fine rhytids and other skin quality issues (e.g., texture, sun-induced damage, pigmentary changes) should be treated with other modalities such as resurfacing (see Chapter 3).

TECHNIQUE

Transconjunctival Lower Blepharoplasty

Transconjunctival blepharoplasty produces less overcorrection than does the transcutaneous approach. It also avoids an external scar. Transcutaneous blepharoplasty frequently alters the lower eyelid margin contour and may cause frank lower eyelid retraction, while only modestly reducing lower skin wrinkles or folds. When redundant skin must be excised, the transconjunctival approach may be combined with anterior skin excision. This will preserve the orbital septum and decrease the risk of postoperative lower eyelid retraction. The transconjunctival approach is the authors' first choice for nearly all patients who are undergoing lower blepharoplasty.

Adequate infiltration of local anesthetic containing epinephrine is critical for patient comfort and hemostasis. Local anesthesia and vasoconstriction is achieved with regional injection of 1 to 2% lidocaine solution containing 1:100,000 epinephrine and hyaluronidase (that is, one vial of hyaluronidase per 50 mL bottle of lidocaine). Bicarbonate may be added to improve the patient's comfort. The conjunctival cul-de-sac is anesthetized with a topical solution prior to injection.

Because the sensory nerves of the conjunctiva and orbital fat originate in the orbit, the injection can effectively be delivered through the conjunctiva. The surgeon directs the needle toward the inferior orbital rim, walks the needle posteriorly until it touches the orbital floor, and then injects approximately 1 mL of anesthetic. The process is repeated to anesthetize each individual fat pocket. The surgeon should allow at least 10 minutes to achieve maximal hemostasis from the epinephrine. Many surgeons prefer to perform lower blepharoplasty with the patient under intravenous sedation. However, the procedure can safely be completed with local anesthesic alone, in selected patients, in the office.

The periorbital region is prepared and draped in sterile, open-face fashion. The drapes should not distort the lower lid–midface contour. The assistant retracts the medial third of the lower eyelid with a small Desmarres retractor to expose the cul-de-sac. A nonconductive eyelid plate may be placed over the globe into the inferior fornix to ballot the globe posteriorly and prolapse orbital fat over the rim.

Conjunctiva and lower lid retractors are incised with a blade or a needle tip directed 1 to 2 mm posterior to the inferior orbital rim (Fig. 2.1). The incision begins at the caruncle and extends laterally toward the lateral canthus. The incision should be made at least 4 mm inferior to the inferior punctum in order to avoid damage to the canaliculus. After the conjunctiva and lower eyelid retractors have been incised, yellow orbital fat bulges into the field. The connective tissue septa may be dissected with the needle tip or with toothed forceps until tufts of fluffy yellow fat are exposed. The assistant removes the glass lid plate and uses 0.5 mm Castroviejo forceps to grasp and lift the lower lid retractors over the globe. This maneuver protects the globe and further prolapses the fat into the field. The Desmarres retractor may be repositioned so that its edge is in the wound itself, thereby providing wider exposure and better visualization of the fat compartments. Placing the connective tissue septa on stretch allows the cutting cautery to expose the fat compartments widely.

Following the primary conjunctival incision, the medial and central fat pads are usually observed first. To improve exposure of the lateral fat pocket, the surgeon often needs to incise the arcuate expansion joining the central fat pad with the lateral fat pad. The lateral fat pad is covered with more septa than the central fat pad, and the fat may not spring forward as easily. After the superficial portion of the lateral fat pad has been excised, the posterior fat comes forward more freely.

The inferior oblique muscle separates the central and medial fat compartments. The surgeon should learn to identify this structure, especially when learning this technique, in order to confirm the identity of the medial fat compartment and to avoid injury to the inferior oblique muscle. Partial resection of the central fat may improve identification of the medial fat. The medial fat appears whiter and more membranous than the fat within the other compartments. Medial prominence of the lower lid primarily represents the medial aspect of the central fat pad rather than a prominent medial fat pad, so care should be taken to avoid excessive medial fat removal.

Meticulous hemostasis is critical during the entire procedure. The blood vessels associated with each fat compartment should be cauterized under direct visualization. Excision is carried out in a graded fashion with the monopolar cautery instrument, incisional laser,

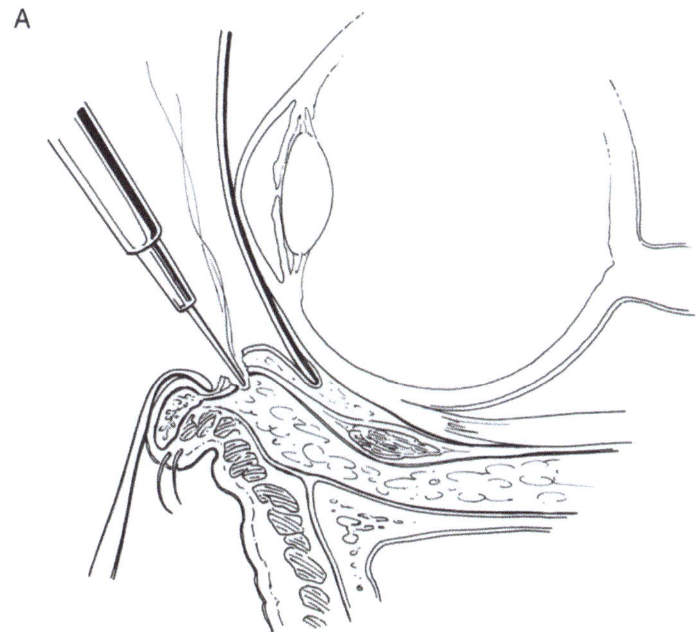

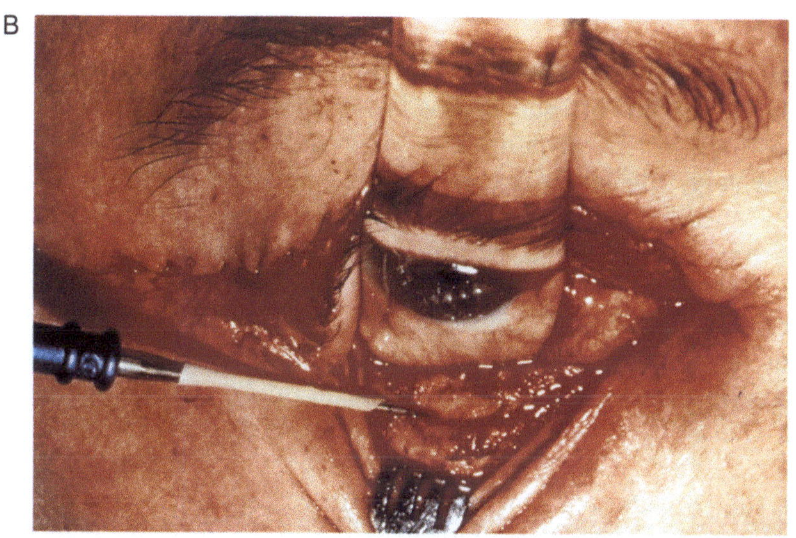

FIGURE 2.1. (A) Line drawing illustrates that the orbital fat may be accessed through the conjunctiva and lower eyelid retractors without violating the orbital septum. (Reproduced with permission from Eyelid surgery. Transconjunctival lower blepharoplasty. In: Nesi FA, Gladstone GJ, Brazzo BG, et al., eds. *Ophthalmic and Facial Plastic Surgery: A Compendium of Reconstructive and Aesthetic Techniques*. Thorofare, NJ: Slack Incorporated, 2000:215.) (B) Surgical photograph demonstrates incision of the conjunctiva and lower eyelid retractors.

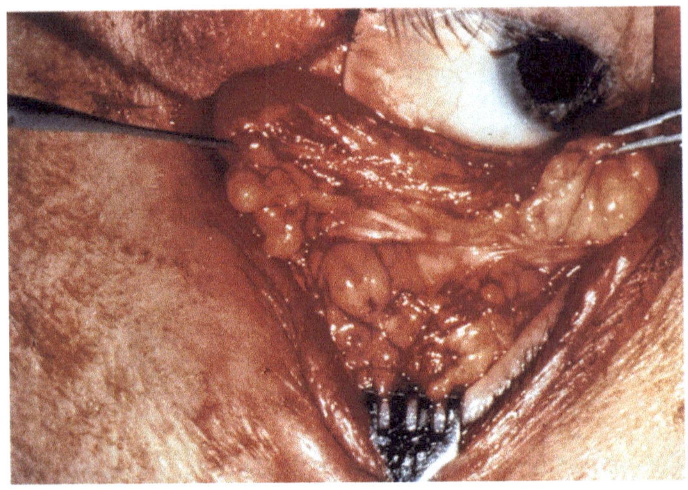

FIGURE 2.2. Fat is excised from each compartment in graded fashion. The endpoint of fat excision is reached when a slight concavity of the lower eyelid exists in the supine position.

scissors, or a blade (Fig. 2.2). The palpebral vessels travel directly through the medial fat pad in the lower eyelid. Meticulous attention to hemostasis in this area should be carried out prior to closure. Intraoperatively, the lower lid is redraped and the contour examined. A slight concavity of the lower lid signifies that the endpoint of fat excision has been reached. Slight pressure on the globe, to simulate upright posture, should restore a single, smooth contour from the eyelid margin to the orbital rim.

After fat removal, the surgeon pulls the lower lid margin superiorly to realign the tissue planes. With the lid on stretch, gentle pressure on the globe reveals any residual fat bulges. If necessary, further fat may be excised. In the author's experience, it is not necessary to close the conjunctiva and lower eyelid retractors; however, two or three interrupted 6-0 absorbable sutures may be used to close the conjunctiva if the tissues do not appear to be well opposed.

Transcutaneous Lower Blepharoplasty

Local anesthesia is performed in a fashion similar to the transconjunctival approach with the addition of approximately 2 mL of the same solution injected transcutaneously within the orbicularis muscle. Sterile preparation with open-face draping is then completed.

                                          Lower Blepharoplasty

It is important to place the lower eyelid incision approximately 2 mm inferior to the lashes. If the incision is placed too close to the lash line, an unnatural crease may occur. The infraciliary incision begins several millimeters temporal to the punctum and follows the lid margin toward the lateral canthus. This incision is created with a #15 Band–Parker blade and extends laterally toward the orbital rim in a preexisting rhytid. When performing quadrilateral blepharoplasty, the surgeon should keep the lateral aspect of the lower lid incision approximately 6 mm inferior to the upper incision to prevent lymphatic flow obstruction. The lateral extent of the lower eyelid incision depends on the amount of skin resection necessary, but usually it ends near the lateral orbital rim.

A 4 mm skin flap is created by undermining inferiorly, along the entire extent of the incision. The preseptal orbicularis muscle is preserved to minimize lower eyelid sphincter damage. Minimal cautery of the underlying orbicularis should be employed to minimize damage to the nutrient supply under the advancement flap of skin. The orbicularis muscle is incised approximately 4 mm inferior to the cutaneous incision and bluntly dissected from the underlying orbital septum (Fig. 2.3). The orbital septum is incised along the entire extent of the eyelid, which allows the redundant orbital fat to bulge into the field.

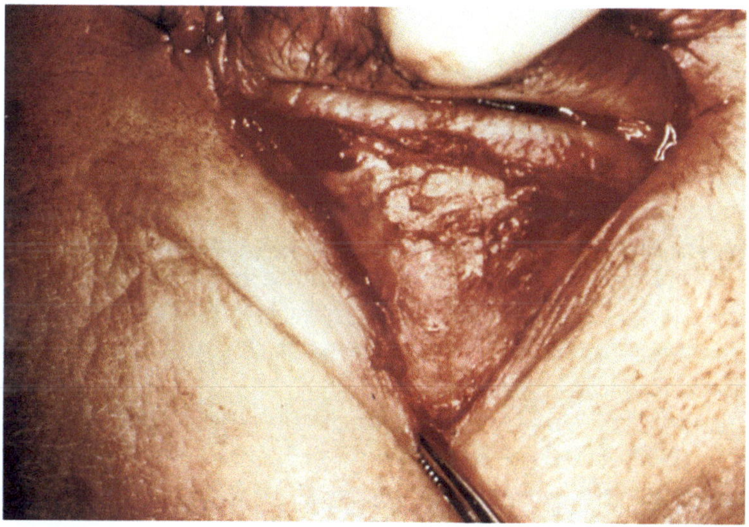

FIGURE 2.3. Surgical photograph demonstrates the orbital septum in relation to the orbicularis. The preserved strip of pretarsal orbicularis muscle allows adequate postoperative sphincter function.

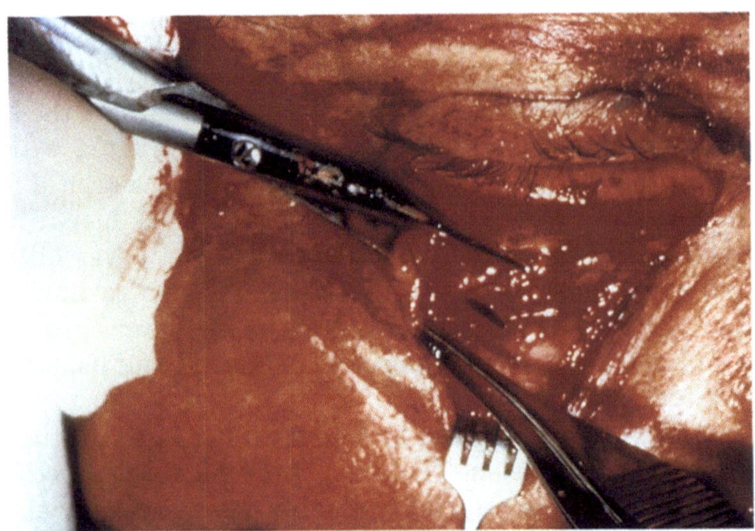

FIGURE 2.4. Graded removal of orbital fat may be performed with scissors. Meticulous hemostasis is achieved with the monopolar cautery instrument.

The thin septa dividing the orbital fat are divided with scissors, monopolar cautery, or incisional laser. Gentle pressure on the globe aids in exposing the redundant fat. The surgeon should minimize traction on the orbital fat to avoid inadvertent hemorrhage. The fat is removed with monopolar cautery, laser, scissors (Fig. 2.4), or a blade, and hemostasis is achieved by cauterization under direct visualization. Although the relative amount of fat to be removed in each of the three fat pockets is determined preoperatively, the surgeon frequently redrapes the skin–muscle flap to check the contour intraoperatively. Care is taken to avoid the inferior oblique muscle, which passes between the medial and central fat compartments. Cauterization of the orbital septum should be avoided because it could lead to postoperative cicatricial eyelid retraction.

The previously undermined skin is redraped over the lower eyelid. The patient is asked to look upward and open the mouth while the surgeon gently ballots the globe to stretch the redraped skin. These maneuvers decrease the risk of excessive skin removal. The amount of redundant skin will be superior to the infraciliary incision, and may be excised by using Stevens scissors or a blade (Fig. 2.5). The cutaneous incision is repaired with interrupted or running absorbable or nonabsorbable suture.

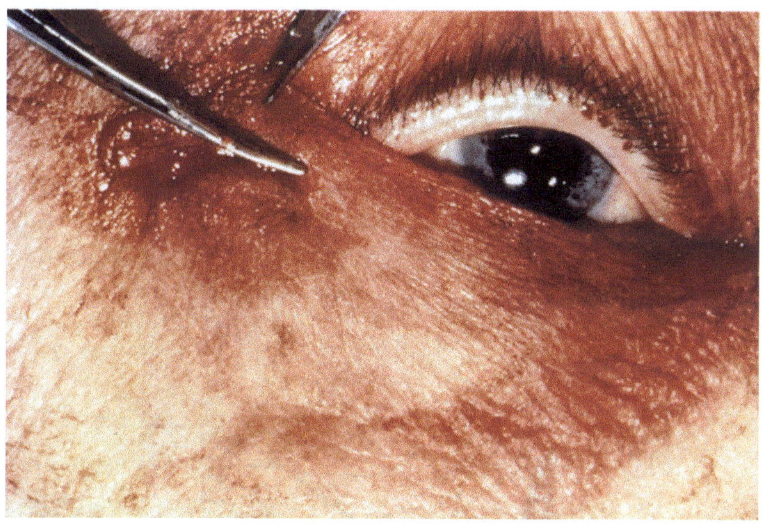

FIGURE 2.5. After the skin flap has been redraped, scissors are used to excise excess eyelid skin.

Avoidance and Repair of Eyelid Laxity

Many patients undergoing lower eyelid skin excision will develop some degree of retraction or ectropion. All patients undergoing transcutaneous lower eyelid fat excision with violation of the orbital septum will develop some degree of lower eyelid retraction. With special precautions, the amount of lower eyelid malposition may be acceptable.

Intraoperatively, a strip of pretarsal orbicularis muscle should be preserved, and manipulation of the orbital septum should be minimized. Only the truly redundant skin should be excised; the previously described intraoperative maneuvers designed to stretch the redraped skin before excision should be employed for every patient undergoing skin excision. Removal of only 2 to 3 mm of skin, followed by application of light cautery for hemostasis, may produce a significant defect when redraped. The preoperative evaluation should identify patients with preexisting lower eyelid laxity, and the surgical plan should be adjusted accordingly.

In patients undergoing lower eyelid skin excision who have little or no horizontal eyelid laxity, concomitant lateral canthal tightening (Webster suture) may decrease the chance of significant postoperative lower eyelid malposition. The lateral canthal tendon is grasped with toothed forceps and advanced laterally until the desired horizontal tension in the lower eyelid is achieved. This will be the amount of lateral canthal tendon that is plicated.

An absorbable suture on a small half-circle needle is used to engage the medial aspect of the inferior crus of the lateral canthal tendon. If significant laxity is present, the suture may need to engage the lateral end of the tarsal plate. The suture then plicates the lateral canthal tendon by affixing the medial aspect of the tendon (or tarsus) to the inner aspect of the lateral orbital rim periosteum in the area of Whitnall's tubercle (Fig. 2.6). A variation of this suture incorporating a small amount of the common crus of the tendon is shown later (Fig. 10.6).

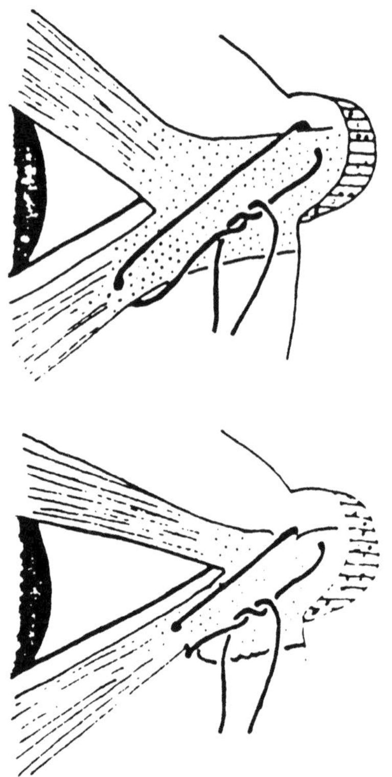

FIGURE 2.6. A lateral canthal plication (Webster) suture provides postoperative support for the lower eyelid and decreases the likelihood of postoperative retraction in patients undergoing transcutaneous lower blepharoplasty with little or no preexisting horizontal laxity. (Reproduced with permission from Classification and treatment of eyelid malposition. In: Nesi FA, Gladstone JG, Brazzo BG, et al., eds. *Ophthalmic and Facial Plastic Surgery: A Compendium of Aesthetic and Reconstructive Techniques.* Thorofare, NJ: Slack Incorporated, 2001:94.)

In all patients undergoing lower eyelid skin excision who have moderate to severe lower eyelid laxity, a concomitant lateral canthal resuspension should be performed to decrease postoperative lower lid malposition.

Postoperative Care

Antibiotic ointment is applied to the wounds and in the eyes at the conclusion of the procedure. Patients are given acetaminophen (650 mg) with or without oxycodone (5 mg) for pain relief. The patient stabilizes in the recovery room for approximately one hour to permit observation for signs of hemorrhage. Upon discharge, patients are cautioned to call the surgeon immediately if severe pain, bleeding, swelling, or decreased vision develops. They are instructed to apply ice packs as often as possible for 2 days following surgery. On the third postoperative day, warm compresses for 15 minutes, four times per day, are instituted. Antibiotic ointment is applied to the wounds and conjunctival cul-de-sac as appropriate. Patients return the following week for suture removal and evaluation.

COMPLICATIONS

Postoperative hemorrhage with resulting blindness is the most feared complication following lower blepharoplasty. While bleeding may occur within the fat compartments, orbicularis bleeding can lead to hematoma formation as well. The patient may complain of severe pain and decreased visual acuity. Examination reveals a firm orbit, proptosis, and subconjunctival hemorrhage associated with decreased vision and an afferent pupillary defect.

Staged treatment is instituted immediately, based on the severity of the hemorrhage and the degree of visual compromise. First, the wound is opened, and blood clots are evacuated. If the signs of orbital compression persist, the lateral canthal tendon is immediately lysed. As a last resort, surgical orbital decompression may allow increased arterial perfusion pressure to the eye and optic nerve. The risk of postoperative hemorrhage can be minimized by meticulous attention to hemostasis intraoperatively, avoiding traction of the fat pedicles during excision, and discontinuing all anticoagulants prior to surgery.

Postoperative cicatricial lower eyelid retraction represents a far more common complication than orbital hemorrhage. This is most commonly the result of excessive surgical injury to the orbital septum, and manifests as lagophthalmos with associated corneal exposure (Fig. 2.7). Treatment of postblepharoplasty cicatricial lower eyelid retraction is discussed in Chapters 9 and 10.

Prevention of this complication requires detailed presurgical evaluation and planning. If skin is removed and no horizontal lower eyelid laxity exists, the authors typically perform lateral canthal plication at the time of skin excision. If frank lower eyelid laxity exists, as determined by the snapback and distraction tests, then concomitant lateral canthal resuspension should be performed. Surgical technique may also help prevent lower eyelid retraction. In the past, surgeons advocated creating a "dog ear" inferiorly as the lower lid incision progressed laterally. This predisposes to lower lid retraction. If lower eyelid incision is extended toward the lateral orbital rim, it should proceed in a horizontal fashion. Leaving a strip of intact pretarsal orbicularis muscle will preserve sphincter function and decrease the risk of postoperative lower eyelid retraction.

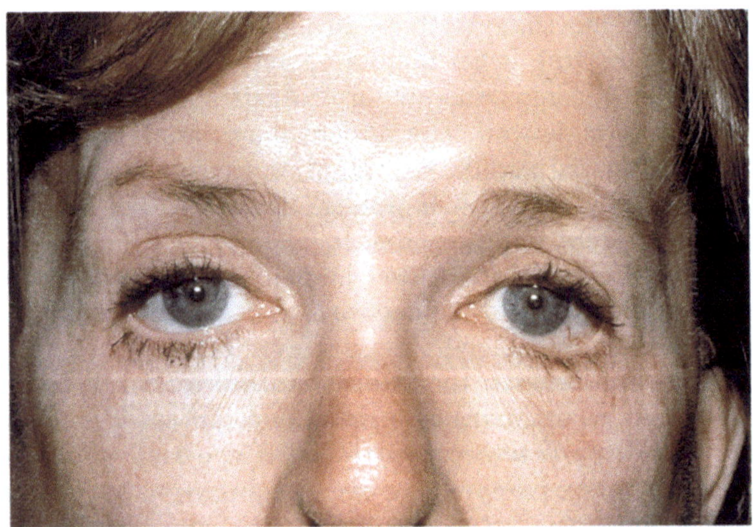

FIGURE 2.7. Following transcutaneous lower blepharoplasty, this patient developed full-thickness vertical inadequacy and lower eyelid retraction.

Other eyelid malpositions may develop after lower blepharoplasty. Ectropion may develop after excessive anterior lamella excision. This complication can be prevented if the surgeon asks the patient to look superiorly and open the mouth, while the surgeon ballots the globe before excising skin. Careful attention to technique should prevent postoperative eyelid malposition.

If the lateral canthal tendon remains lax in the postoperative period, the patient is at higher risk of developing eyelid retraction or ectropion. In some cases, if one tendon becomes dehisced, eyelid asymmetry may appear, and one palpebral fissure may appear smaller than the other (Fig. 2.8). Repositioning of the canthal tendon with lateral tarsal strip procedure will correct the imbalance.

Unsightly cutaneous scarring may occur after transcutaneous blepharoplasty. If the incision is placed too close or too distant from the lashes, the infraciliary scar may be more noticeable. When the incision is carried laterally, it should not be directed downward, as depicted in some older texts. This may result in a scar running perpendicular to the relaxed skin tension lines. If simultaneous upper blepharoplasty is performed, the upper incision should be at least

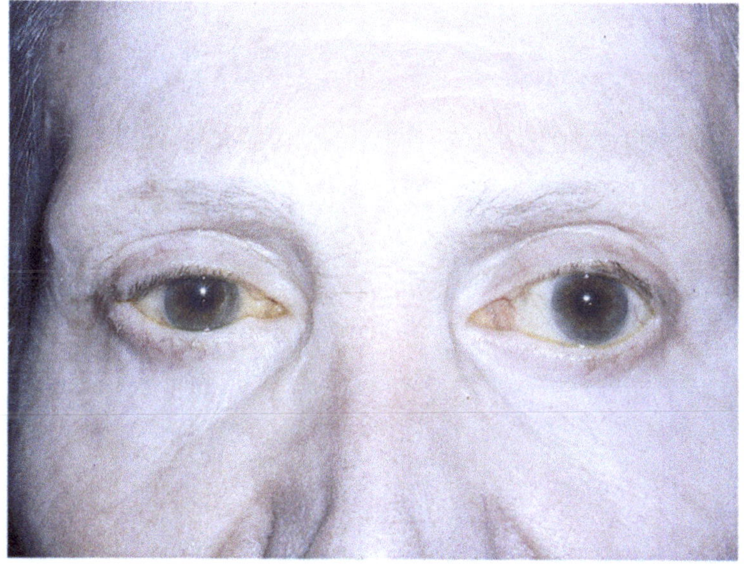

FIGURE 2.8. Several years following transcutaneous blepharoplasty, this patient requested repair of eyelid asymmetry. She had complete right lateral canthal tendon dehiscence, which was repaired with lateral tarsal strip.

6 to 7 mm superior to the lower incision in the lateral canthal area to avoid persistent lymphedema.

Occasionally, too much or too little fat is removed or repositioned. This complication can be minimized by frequent intraoperative redraping and assessment. Despite what the surgeon believes to be an adequate postoperative result, a patient may be dissatisfied. Typically, this occurs when a physician who did not understand the underlying concepts unknowingly offered unrealistic expectations to a patient. A detailed knowledge of the underlying anatomy, the concept that lower blepharoplasty will not treat skin texture abnormalities, and knowledge of the lower eyelid–midface anatomical continuum should prevent this unfortunate complication.

3

LASER RESURFACING

- Michael Mercandetti
- Adam J. Cohen

The use of lasers to reduce the effects of age and photo-related damage to facial skin has gained widespread acceptance. Initially the carbon dioxide (CO_2), then the erbium: yttrium–aluminum–garnet (Er:YAG), and more recently the combined CO_2/erbium lasers offer wavelengths and fluences that produce clinically significant and controlled cutaneous exfoliation with a limited surrounding injury zone.

The wavelengths (10,600 nm for the CO_2 laser and 2940 nm for the erbium laser) are highly absorbed by water, which is the chromophore. Water constitutes 72% of skin volume. The erbium wavelength is absorbed by water approximately 16 times greater than is CO_2 wavelength.[1]

Although the outcomes of cutaneous laser surgery are often excellent (Fig. 3.1), complications arise. Several preoperative, intraoperative, and postoperative considerations are paramount in decreasing complication rates.

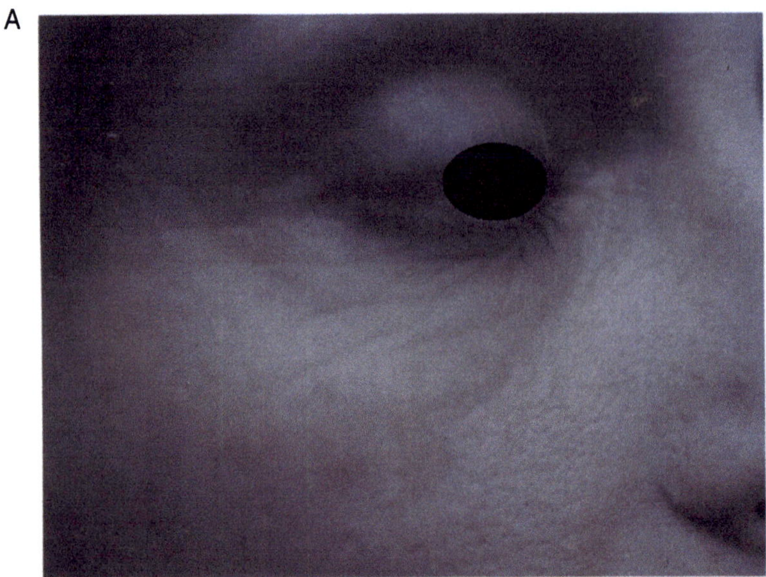

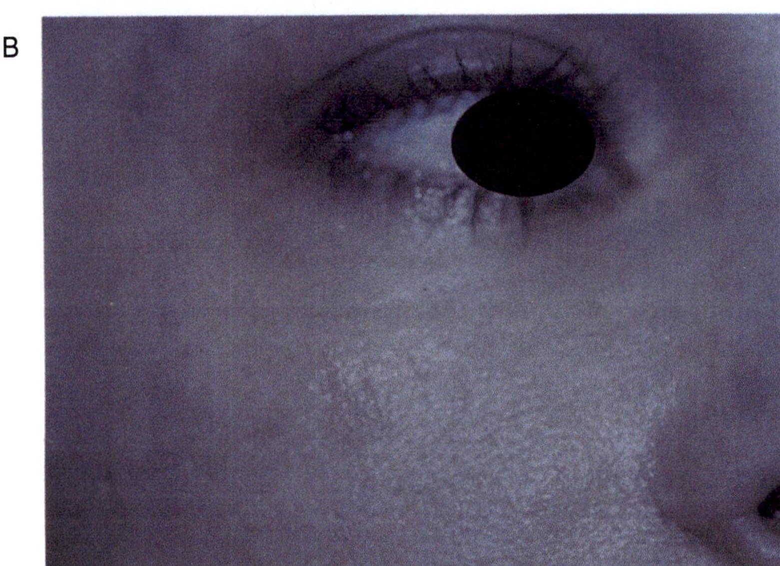

FIGURE 3.1. (A) Lateral and infraorbital rhytids prior to treatment with the erbium laser. (B) Reduction in rhytids following complete healing.

EVALUATION

Potential sources of complications can sometimes be identified during the prelaser evaluation. As with any procedure, a detailed medical and dermatological history with emphasis on wound healing and scar formation is essential. A thorough history of abnormal wound healing, skin disorders, and ethnic background can influence the outcome.

If the patient has a history of collagen vascular diseases (e.g., lupus), keloid formation, or immunological abnormalities (e.g., vitiligo), laser treatment should be avoided. These conditions can result in serious healing problems.

A history of isotretinoin (Accutane) use within the year prior to laser resurfacing is a contraindication to resurfacing. The epithelium of the adnexal structures is a source of cells for reepithelization of the lasered skin. Accutane and facial radiation, which has been used in the past for treatment of acne and enlargement of the thyroid gland, inhibit these adnexal structures. The authors highly recommend pretreating a small area and assessing the healing response before proceeding with a full treatment. The newer nonablative lasers such as the frequency-modified Nd:YAG, the broadband high-intensity pulsed light, and the flashlamp dye laser appear to affect the dermal collagen without the exfoliative process. These lasers may be less risky in these patients, since the epidermis is not removed.

The surgeon should consider the support of the mimetic muscles and position of overlying soft tissues, which can contribute to facial, midfacial, and neck ptosis. In certain patients the required skin tightening and rhytid reduction cannot be achieved with laser alone. Instead facelift, midface lift, forehead elevation, or blepharoplasty may need to be performed alone or in conjunction with laser.

If a patient is undergoing an endoscopic forehead lift or a transconjunctival blepharoplasty, combined laser resurfacing can be performed safely. In these procedures, the tissues retain adequate vascularity. If the lid surgeries are done with a transcutaneous approach, the authors do not resurface concomitantly. Instead, the tissue is allowed to heal, and resurfacing can be done approximately 4 weeks afterward.

The patient's degree of pigmentation plays an extremely important role in laser resurfacing. This consideration involves the patient's normal or "baseline" pigment, as well as acquired pigmentation from sun exposure or other conditions, including melasma. Patients with darker skin types exhibit a higher incidence of both hyperpigmentation and hypopigmentation. Conversely, extremely light-skinned patients may be more prone to develop prolonged erythema postoperatively. Hormonal changes during pregnancy can vary the amount of pigmentation, and resurfacing in women who are pregnant is contraindicated.

The authors differentiate patients who are Fitzpatrick class I and II (light pigmentation) from the other classes. The class I and II patients are "prepped" for 2 weeks prior to surgery by using 10% glycolic acid twice a day and Renova (tretinoin emollient cream 0.05%, Ortho Pharmaceutical Corp., Raritan, NJ) at bedtime. The 10% glycolic acid is either of the MD Forté line (Allergan; Irvine, CA) or Dermatopix (Pharmagen; Bohemia, NY). The latter is supplied in easy-to-use circular cotton-type pads impregnated with the glycolic acid.

Some surgeons, however, feel that preoperative treatment with retinoic acids can contribute to postoperative erythema. If a patient has had problems with Renova, the authors substitute Kinerase (N^6-furfuryladenine, 0.1%, ICN Pharmaceuticals; Costa Mesa, CA).

Additionally, a bleaching agent may be added. Typically the authors recommend lotion containing 4% hydroquinone from the Dermatopix or Obagi line products (Obagi Medical Products; Long Beach, CA). The 4% hydroquinone can also be obtained from ICN Pharmaceuticals, which manufactures Solaquin Forté cream and gel (both of which contain sunscreens), Eldopaque Forté cream with sunblock, and Eldoquin Forté cream without sunscreen or sunblock (ICN Pharmaceuticals). There are other hydroquinones such as Lustra (Medicis Pharmaceutical Corp.; Phoenix, AZ) and Melenex, which is 3% hydroquinone (Neutrogena Corp.; Los Angeles), both of which are available with a prescription. Patients treated with these products are also treated with tretinoin (Retin-A, Geneva Pharmaceuticals, Inc., Broomfield, CO).

For patients of Fitzpatrick class III and IV, the regimen is started 4 weeks prior to treatment. For all patients, hypoallergenic sunscreen rated at least SPF-15 is recommended. All patients need to understand that they must to avoid sun exposure, particularly in the postoperative period.

A recent study indicated that preoperative treatment using either 10% glycolic acid or 4% hydroquinone and 0.025% retinoic acid did

Laser Resurfacing

not affect postoperative hyperpigmentation in patients (Fitzpatrick classes I–III).[2] The reason is that the epidermal melanocytes, which are affected by these agents, are destroyed by the laser process and therefore do not contribute to the pigmentary changes. This topic continues to be debated by laser experts.

If a patient has a history of facial herpetic disease, pretreatment with antiviral medicine such as acyclovir, famciclovir, or valacyclovir should be considered, particularly if the perioral area will be treated. The authors currently use famciclovir (500 mg po, bid), starting the day of the treatment and continuing for 10 days. If the patient does not have a history of herpetic outbreaks and is having perioral laser, the authors pretreat the patient. If the patient has no history of a herpetic outbreak and no treatment of the perioral area is planned, prophylaxis is not recommended. All patients are given antibiotic pretreatment, usually cephalexin (Keflex, 250 mg po, qid for 10 days) or cefuroxime (Ceftin, 250 mg po bid for 10 days). If the patient has a penicillin allergy, doxycycline (100 mg po bid) or ciprofloxacin (250 mg po bid) for 10 days is a reasonable alternative.[3–5]

Many patients are concerned about lifestyle considerations and recovery. If a patient anticipates being back at work in a few days, then laser resurfacing might not be appropriate. Even a low-fluence erbium treatment will require recovery time. For these patients, other modalities such as particle resurfacing (microdermabrasion), glycolic peels, low-strength trichloracetic acid (TCA) peels, or the nonablative laser and light treatments can be considered. However, the degree of rhytid reduction will not equal that of the laser, and the patient must be made aware of this compromise.

No matter how skilled the surgeon, one must remember that the patient's psychosocial state and expectations affect the perceived outcome. A clinically satisfactory endpoint can be achieved in the eyes of the surgeon but not the patient. Therefore it is prudent to address all concerns of the patient, designating the anatomical areas to be addressed, and to clearly explain and document the discussion of what can and cannot be accomplished by the procedure.

Once the determination to proceed with laser resurfacing has been made, different lasers are available. Depending on the clinical practice CO_2, erbium, combined CO_2/erbium, or pulse-duration-modified erbium might be available. The authors have greatest experience with the CO_2 and erbium lasers. Initially the CO_2 laser was used in all cases, because it was the only one available. When the erbium laser

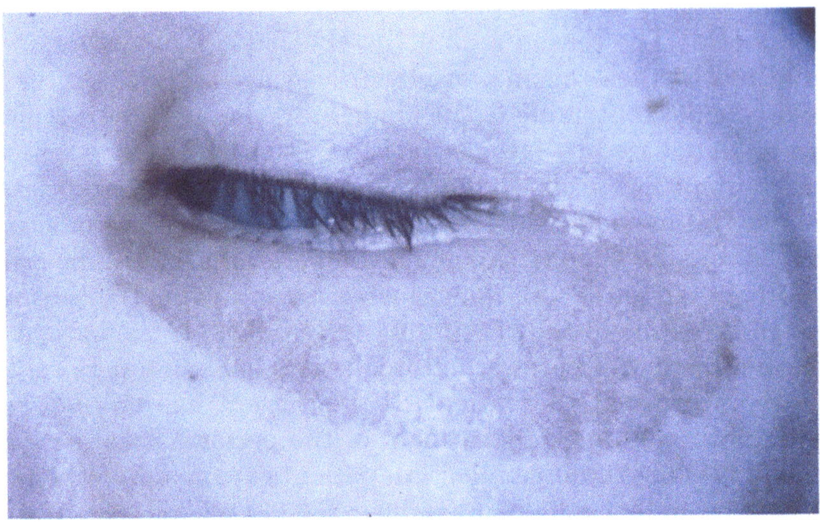

FIGURE 3.2. A patient immediately after treatment using the CO_2 laser. To produce an appropriate response, the laser must ablate the epidermis and some of the papillary dermis without breaching the deeper dermis.

became available, different protocols were followed. The younger patients who had fewer and shallower rhytids, and the patients who had more pigment, were treated with the erbium. The older patients who had deeper rhytids were treated with the CO_2 laser.

The authors believe that even older patients, with deeper rhytids, can be successfully treated with the erbium laser, but higher fluence is required and the healing time is longer, although still less than that of the CO_2 laser.[6] Faster healing follows treatment with the erbium[7], particularly when low fluence is used on shallow rhytids. When higher fluence is applied, healing time tends to be longer.[8] The effect of the laser on dermal collagen tightening must also be considered. Patients treated with the CO_2 laser will more likely experience significant collagen remodeling and tightening, while those treated with the erbium laser will experience only wound contracture secondary to tissue healing.[9]

Laser Resurfacing

TECHNIQUE

The surgeon should have a clear and thorough understanding of laser applications and techniques and should be cognizant of how the laser parameters will affect outcome. The surgeon must use power settings that achieve a suitable radiant energy to conductive heat ratio, allowing for optimal surgical results[10] (Fig. 3.2).

The American National Standards Institute (ANSI) establishes the national standards for the safe operation of lasers. The Occupational Safety and Health Administration (OSHA) also has guidelines that must be adhered to by all personnel involved in the use of lasers.

As a result, protective eye shields are required for the patient and protective eyewear for all personnel. A protective mouth guard is to be used by the patient who is having perioral treatment with the erbium laser, which can burn enamel. Instruments and protectors used on the patient should be of a dulled metal variety. Plastic eyeshields are not to be used because either CO_2 or erbium laser can burn through the plastic. Areas that are not to be treated should be protected with dull foil or wet towels. Laser goggles used by personnel involved in the operation should be wavelength appropriate and of an optical density high enough to afford adequate protection.

A high-quality smoke evacuator is essential to reduce the plume created by the laser treatment. Human papillomavirus has been recovered from smoke plume. Laser filtration masks that filter out particles at least 1 μm in diameter with a 95% or higher efficiency should be used.

There is risk of the laser igniting supplementary oxygen, and therefore appropriate precautions are required. If the patient is under general anesthesia, additional protection is needed to avoid lasering the intubation tube and igniting the flammable gases. Special laser-resistant tubes are available. Skin preps should be nonflammable.

The surgeon and the technician must jointly verify the laser settings. The laser should be tested prior to use to ensure its proper functioning. Depending on the laser used, the area to be treated, the degree of rhytidosis, and the amount of pigmentation, the number of passes used will be uniquely determined. Even for the same patient, the number of the passes will vary depending on the area of the face treated.

COMPLICATIONS

The primary postoperative goal is to facilitate healing of the epithelium. Pain, serous discharge, and crusting occur in all cases (Fig. 3.3). Mild bleeding may occur following erbium resurfacing (Figs. 3.4 and 3.5). The decision to cover the skin or leave it "open" postoperatively varies. The authors currently use an open technique, most often utilizing Aquaphor. The patient is advised to keep the skin moist throughout the day and night. A narcotic analgesic should usually be prescribed. If the treatment is to a local area, such as under the eyes, acetaminophen alone may suffice.

The treated area should be kept cool, but not wet, by applying finely crushed, soft ice compresses in 15-minute cycles for 2 to 3 days. Oral steroids are not prescribed. The antibiotic and antiviral regimens are continued for several days. Diphenhydramine (Benadryl) can be recommended for pruritis.

The patient is seen in the office on the first postlaser day. A gentle cleaning is carried out using a mixture of hydrogen peroxide and

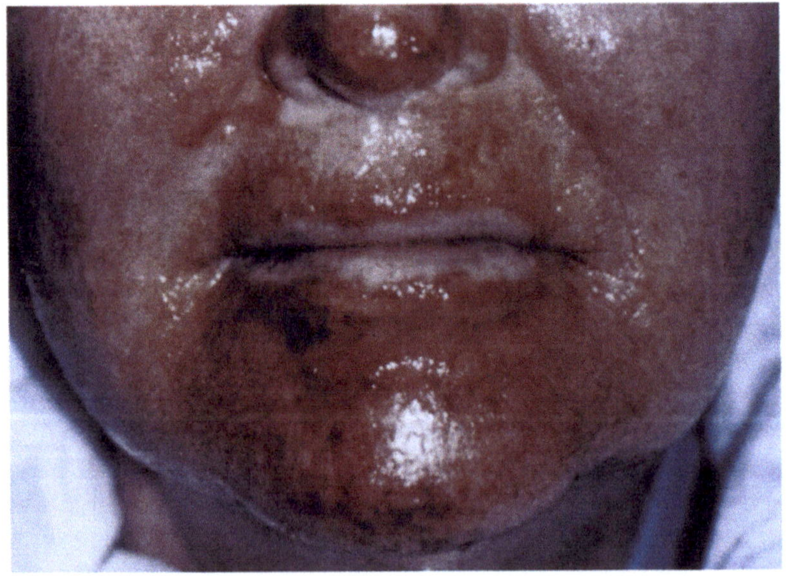

FIGURE 3.3. A patient one day after treatment using the CO_2 laser. The patient's skin was left open and moisturized with Aquaphor.

                                    Laser Resurfacing

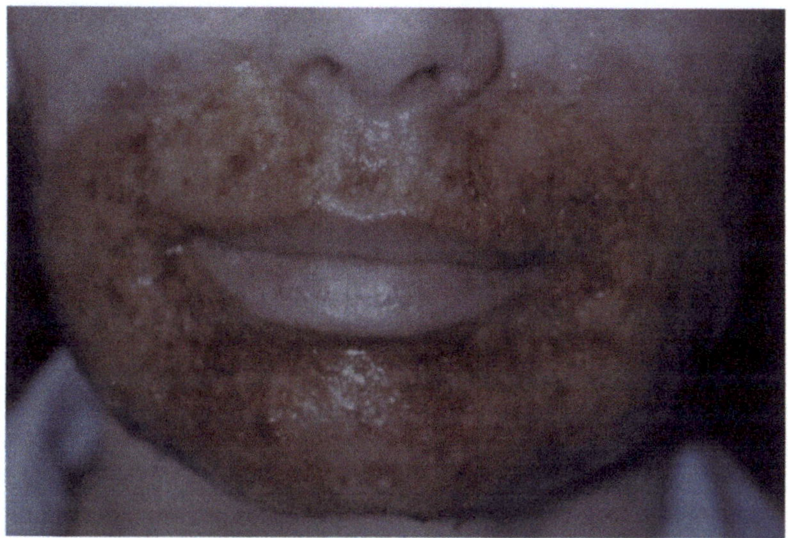

FIGURE 3.4. Normal exudation and crusting of the skin one day posterbium laser. The patient's skin was left open and moisturized with Aquaphor.

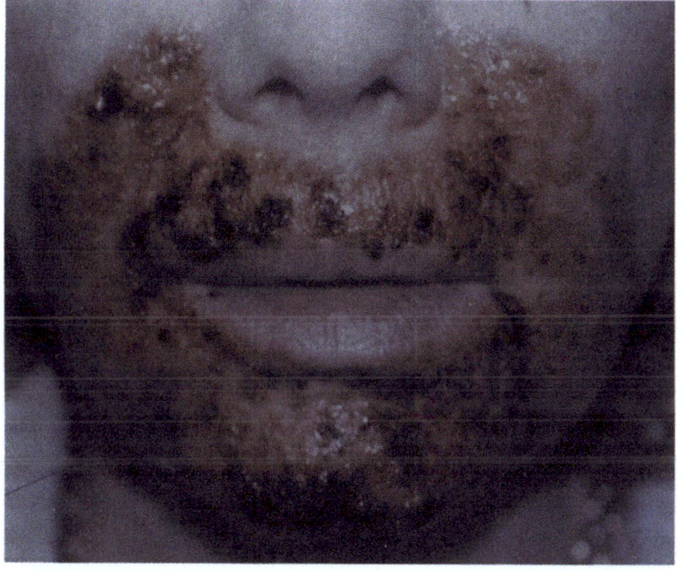

FIGURE 3.5. Normal exudation and crusting of the skin one day posterbium laser. The patient's skin was left open and moisturized with Aquaphor. Note the greater degree of hemorrhagic crusting indicated by the dark crusts.

warm water (1:3 mixture). The aim is to remove as much crusting and debris as possible without initiating bleeding. Erbium-treated skin demonstrates more bleeding if the cleansing is aggressive. The epidermis will regenerate fastest and heal with fewer complications if wounds are kept clean and moist.

The Aquaphor is reapplied and the patient is instructed to maintain this regimen. The authors see the patient again on the fourth to seventh day after the treatment and then weekly. After the skin reepithelizes, the Aquaphor is discontinued.

The daily treatment regimen then consists of gentle facial cleansing using Cetaphil Gentle Skin Cleanser (Gladerma Laboratories, Fort Worth, TX), Aderma Septalibour Ultra Gentle Purifying Cleanser (Pierre Fabre Dermatology, Azusa, CA) or Oil of Olay Sensitive Skin (Procter & Gamble, Cincinnati, OH). The authors also have the patient use sunscreen or sunblock and a bleaching agent (4% hydroquinone, bid). Glyquin from ICN contains 4% hydroquinone, 10% glycolic acid, L-ascorbic acid as stabilizer, and sunscreen. An SPF-65 clear lotion or SPF-60 foundation/cover-up sunblock is available from Fallene (Fallene Ltd., King of Prussia, PA).

The authors highly recommend avoiding exposure to the sun. After the epidermis has healed, camouflage makeup can be used, such as Physicians Formula Self Defense (Physicians Formula Cosmetics, Azusa, CA). After the third or fourth week, 5 to 10% glycolic acid treatment at home can be added. In addition Renova, Retina-A, or Kinerase once every other day for a week and then once a day as tolerated can be used. Patients may use a hypoallergenic, fragrance-free moisturizer throughout the day such as Eucerin Dry Skin Therapy (Beiersdorf Inc., Norwalk, CT) or Almay Time-Off Lasting Moisture (Almay Inc., New York).

The erbium-treated skin reepithelizes faster than CO_2-treated skin, but this can vary depending on the fluences used. During the healing period, the skin is hypersensitive to allergens in the topical preparations and in the air; the incidence of contact dermatitis is high. Topical antibiotics and moisturizers with fragrance are to be avoided because they are more likely to provoke an allergic reaction. Even after the epithelium has healed, the skin remains hypersensitive. Hypoallergenic and fragrance-free soaps should be used because patients are very susceptible to reactions from laundry soaps and fabric softeners even if these products had been used without incident prior to treatment (Fig. 3.6). Milia, which are small white cystic lesions, and acne can occur from occlusive dressings and thick ointments used in the immediate postlaser period.[11]

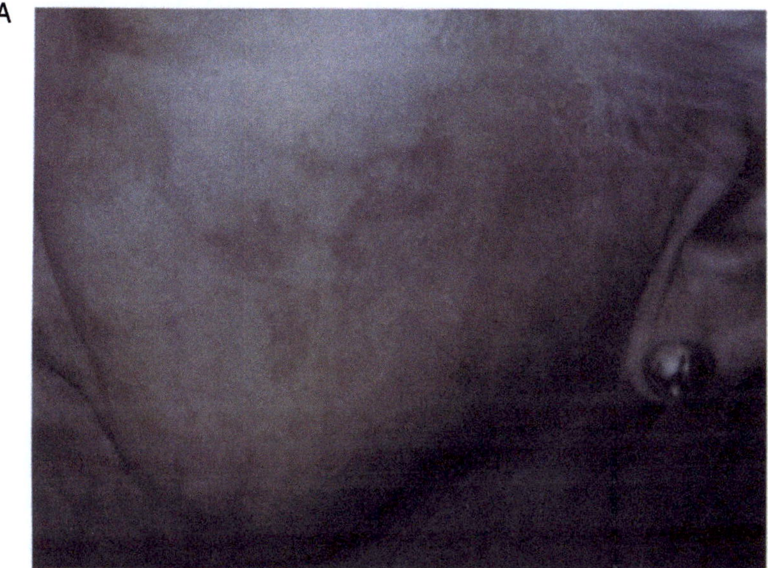

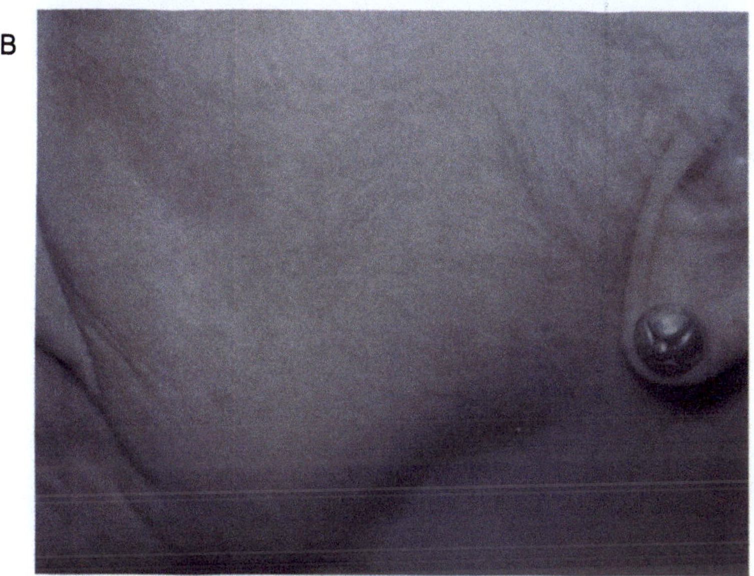

FIGURE 3.6. (A) Contact dermatitis secondary to commercial fabric softener. The patient, who had undergone facial resurfacing with the CO_2 laser, slept on this side of her face. (B) After treatment with steroid cream and cessation of the use of the fabric softener, the dermatitis resolved without sequelae.

Erythema is always seen regardless of which laser is used. Prolonged erythema is often bothersome to patients (Fig. 3.7). Erythema can persist for a few months, and the prolonged inflammation increases the chance of hyperpigmentation (Fig. 3.8). Erythema has been reported to be less with the erbium laser,[7,12] most likely because lower energy is used. Ascorbic acid has been shown to have

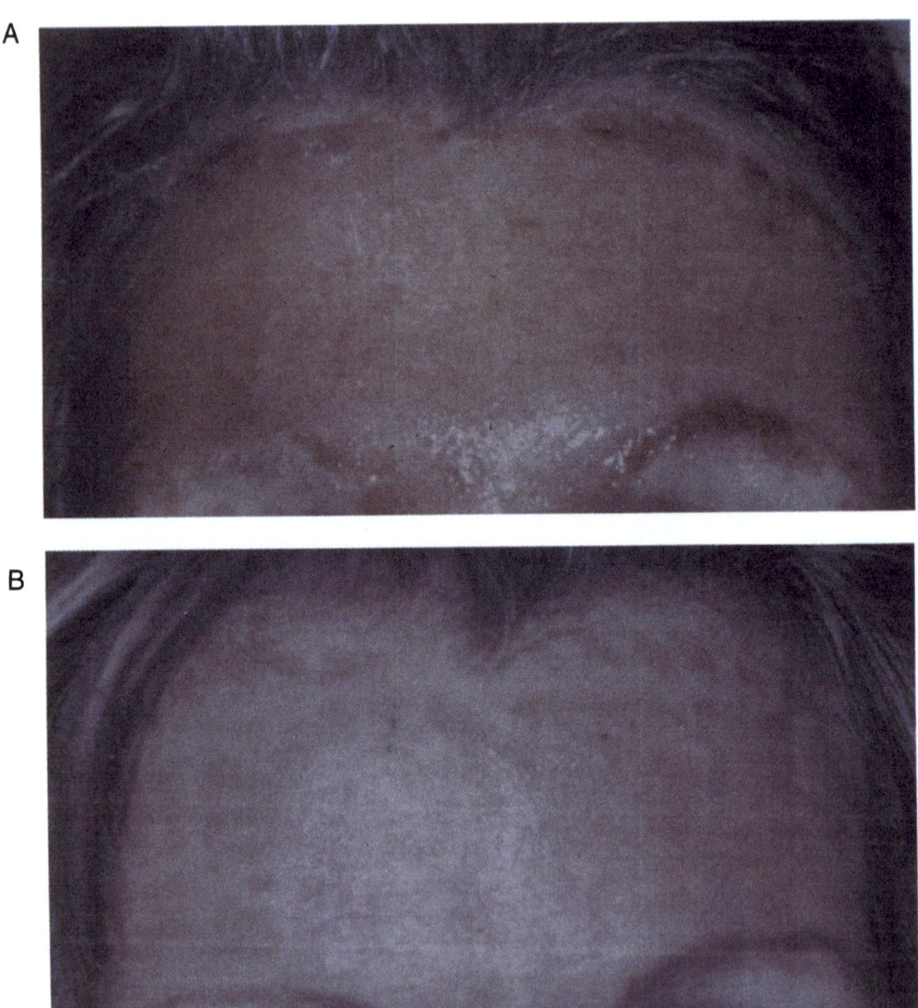

FIGURE 3.7. (A) Forehead of patient one day after treatment with the CO_2 laser. (B) Same patient, 19 days after treatment. The erythema has subsided slowly, but still persists with some hyperpigmentation. Mild blotchiness corresponding to the pattern generator can be noted.

                                                                 Laser Resurfacing

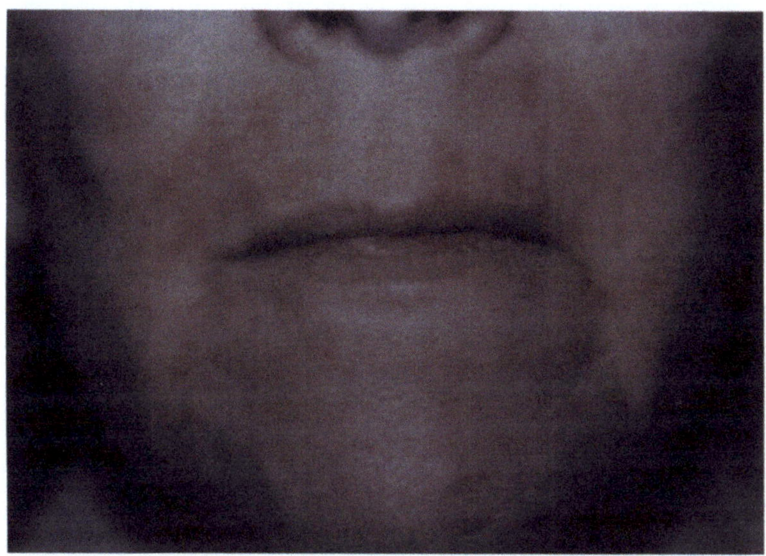

FIGURE 3.8. Perioral erythema and hyperpigmentation, postresurfacing.

anti-inflammatory properties and can be used postoperatively.[13] Steroids, such as 1% hydrocortisone, can be utilized to lessen erythema. Stronger steroids can be used for a short duration to avoid atrophy of the skin. After the epithelium has healed, camouflaging cosmetics are appropriate until the redness has subsided.

Microbial infections usually begin before full reepithelialization is complete. Herpes outbreaks occur in about 2 to 7% of patients who receive antiviral prophylaxis.[14] Since bacterial, viral, or fungal pathogens are all potential etiologies, prompt and accurate diagnosis and aggressive treatment are important to reduce scarring and further dissemination. Many surgeons will prophylactically treat patients with antivirals and antibiotics.[3–5]

Postinflammatory hyperpigmentation usually surfaces approximately 5 weeks after laser surgery. One-third of all patients experience pigmentary changes. This risk is greater in patients with higher melanocyte levels.[9] Pigmentary changes, though usually transient, can be prolonged and quite noticeable. Regimens to reduce the hyperpigmentation include the use of bleaching agents such as hydroquinone, kojic acid, and 20% azelaic acid (Azelex, Allergan), with or without facial glycolic acid or TCA peeling treatments. Care must be taken to avoid inducing erythema with these treatments, which can result in increased hyperpigmentation.

Hypopigmentary changes are usually permanent and manifest several months after resurfacing. This difficult situation can be reduced with skin-colored tattooing, application of makeup, or reduction of the normal surrounding pigmentation with various peeling agents.

Hypertrophic scarring and ectropion are rarely encountered but can be severe complications. Robust scar formation most often follows damage of the adnexa of the lower face and neck. In the early phases, a 585 nm pulsed dye laser can be used to reduce the vascular component of this unsettling sequela.[15] Thickened scars can be treated with high-strength topical or intralesional steroids, silicone gel, silicone sheets, or Mederma (Mederma Skin Care for Scars, Lawrenceville, GA). Keloid formation is an exuberant scarring that extends beyond the borders of the treated area. Keloids are usually treated in a fashion similar to hypertrophic scarring but for a longer period. Keloids may need to be corrected surgically, but the surgeon must be wary of keloid re-formation caused by the surgery itself.

If mild ectropion develops, it can be treated with massage and topical steroids such as 1% hydrocortisone or fluorometholone ointment. For a short course, a stronger steroid, such as 0.05% betamethasone, can also be used. Intralesional steroid injection of triamcinolone diacetate (10 mg/mL) is another option. Again the surgeon should be wary of atrophy and hypopigmentation from steroid use. A temporary tarsorraphy suture can be used. If possible, the surgeon should wait for the scar to mature. However if the ectropion is severe or has not improved despite the treatments recommended, surgical repair should be performed.

Hypotrophic scarring is less commonly encountered. Filler material, such as Collagen (McGhan Medical; Santa Barbara, California), can be used if the hypotrophic scarring is localized.

REFERENCES

1. Walsh JT, Deutsch TF. Er:YAG laser ablation of tissue: measurement of ablation rates. *Lasers Surg Med* 1989;9:327.

2. West TB, Alster TS. Effect of pretreatment on the incidence of hyperpigmentation following cutaneous CO_2 laser resurfacing. *Dermatol Surg* 1999;25:15–17.

3. Sriprachya-Anunt S, Fitzpatrick RE, Goldman MP, Smith SR. Infections complicating pulsed carbon dioxide laser resurfacing for photoaged facial skin. *Dermatol Surg* 1997;23:527–535; Discussion:535–536.

4. Manuskiatti W, Fitzpatrick RE, Goldman MP, Krejci-Papa N. Prophylactic antibiotics in patients undergoing laser resurfacing of the skin. *J Am Acad Dermatol* 1999;40:77–84.

5. Walia S, Alster TS. Cutaneous CO_2 laser resurfacing infection rate with and without prophylactic antibiotics. *Dermatol Surg* 1999;25:857–861.

6. Bass LS, Plastic Surgery Educational Foundation DATA Committee. Skin resurfacing with erbium:YAG lasers. *Plast Reconstr Surg* January 2000;105(1):462–463.

7. Bass LS. Erbium:YAG laser skin resurfacing: preliminary clinical evaluation. *Ann Plast Surg* April 1998;40(4):328–334.

8. Adrian RM. Pulsed carbon dioxide and erbium-YAG laser resurfacing: a comparative clinical and histological study. *J Cutan Laser Ther* 1999;1:29–35.

9. Fitzpatrick RE, Rostan EF, Marchell N. Collagen tightening induced by carbon dioxide laser versus erbium:YAG laser. *Laser Surg Med* 2000;27:395–403.

10. Reid R. Physical and surgical principles governing carbon dioxide laser surgery on the skin. *Dermatol Clin* 1991;9(2):297–316.

11. Nanni CA, Alster TS. Complications of carbon dioxide laser resurfacing. An evaluation of 500 patients. *Dermatol Surg* 1998;24:315.

12. Mercandetti M. Erb:YAG or CO_2 laser treatment of periocular wrinkles: Which is better? Presentation at the American Academy of Ophthalmology Annual Meeting, 1998; Orlando FL.

13. Alster TS, West TB. Effects of topical vitamin C on postoperative carbon dioxide resurfacing erythema. *Dermatol Surg* 1998;24:331.

14. Alster TS, Nanni CA. Famcyclovir prophylaxis of herpes simplex virus: reactivation after laser resurfacing. *Dermatol Surg* 1999;25:3.

15. Alster TS. Improvement of erythematous and hypertrophic scars by the 585 nm flashlamp-pumped pulsed dye laser. *Ann Plast Surg* 1994;32:186–190.

BIBLIOGRAPHY

Alster TS. Laser resurfacing of rhytids. In: Alster TS, ed. *Manual of Cutaneous Laser Techniques*. Philadelphia: Lippincott-Raven; 1997:104.

Fitzpatrick RE. Facial resurfacing with the pulsed carbon dioxide laser: a review. *Facial Plast Surg Clin North Am* 1996;4(2):231.

Jacobson D, Bass LS, VanderKam V, Achauer, BM. Carbon dioxide and Er:YAG laser resurfacing. Results. *Clin Plast Surg* April 2000;27(2):241–250.

Walsh JT, Flotte TJ, Anderson RR, et al. Pulsed CO_2 laser tissue ablation: effect of tissue type and pulse duration on thermal damage. *Lasers Surg Med* 1988;8:108.

4

FOREHEAD LIFT

• Brian G. Brazzo

The eyebrows and forehead are distinct features of the face. When aesthetically pleasing, they can convey a sense of restfulness, attractiveness, and health. However, with drooping of the eyebrows and contraction of the frontalis muscle, the upper face may appear sad, tired, or angry. Furthermore, a sagging forehead can create heavy upper eyelids, brow ache, and functional eyelid problems.

The goals of rejuvenation surgery of the brow and upper forehead include elevation of drooping eyebrows, reduction of excess upper lid skin, elevation of the forehead, reduction of forehead wrinkles, softening of lateral crow's feet, and correction of eyebrow asymmetry. Aesthetic goals of upper face rejuvenation are different for men and women. Successful forehead lifts require a complete understanding of aesthetic facial proportions as they pertain to each sex. Brow elevation should be conservative, and the brows should not be overly arched in men. Some men feel their forehead lines convey a sense of power, masculinity, and authority. When undertaking a browlift, one may choose to attenuate these wrinkles without completely eradicating them as in women. Before forehead rejuvenation, a careful evaluation of brow position and contour, forehead wrinkles, hairline, and upper eyelids is essential, and surgeon and patient must agree on the goals of the procedure.

EVALUATION

• Jessica Lattman

A visually pleasing eyebrow is considerably different in men and women. To begin with, men and women differ anatomically. The male eyebrow is heavier, less arched, and lower than that of the female. The space between the eyelashes and the brow is typically smaller in a male than in a female, with a lower position of the eyebrow. Furthermore, the skin around the male eyebrow is thicker and contains more sweat glands. The male forehead is also wider and the orbicularis oculi, frontalis, procerus, and corrugator are heavier, resulting in deeper furrows and more pronounced crows'-feet.

The evaluation of ptosis, dermatochalasis, and eyebrow ptosis are covered in Chapters 6 to 8. For patients with true brow ptosis, several factors assist the surgeon in predicting which ones will respond best to endoscopic forehead lift. One concept is "frame height," the distance from the center of the pupil to the top of the brow. If this distance is less than 2.0 to 2.5 cm, then brow ptosis is likely present and forehead lift is indicated.

The "glide test" measures the distance an examiner or patient can lift the brow from its resting position. Measurements may be taken from medial, central, and lateral brow points and averaged. Older patients with frame heights between 1.5 to 2.0 cm and with glide tests between 2 to 3 cm tend to do well with endoscopic brow elevation.

Before surgery, the authors recommend that patients stop smoking. Cigarettes can inhibit healing and decrease blood supply to the skin. This is especially important in men, who are at increased risk for bleeding given their thicker, more vascular skin. All aspirin, ibuprofen, and other blood-thinning medications (Coumadin, vitamin E, homeopathic medications) should be stopped in consultation with the patient's internist. Some vitamin supplements are believed to aid the healing process and minimize bruising. These include vitamin C and vitamin K, which may be taken before surgery. Coffee and other caffeine-containing products should be avoided the night before surgery.

Many different surgical techniques now exist, each with its benefits, difficulties, and suitability for a specific situation. The forehead can be surgically lifted through several approaches: endoscopic, coronal, midforehead, direct brow, and internal brow (browpexy, through a blepharoplasty incision). A newer, nonsurgical approach to upper face rejuvenation is the use of botulinum toxin (Botox) to smooth forehead wrinkles and slightly elevate the medial eyebrow.

TECHNIQUES

Endoscopic Forehead Lift

The endoscopic technique for forehead lifting was first described in 1991, and since then has gained wide acceptance. When using an endoscope (Fig. 4.1), which is a miniature lighted telescope, the sur-

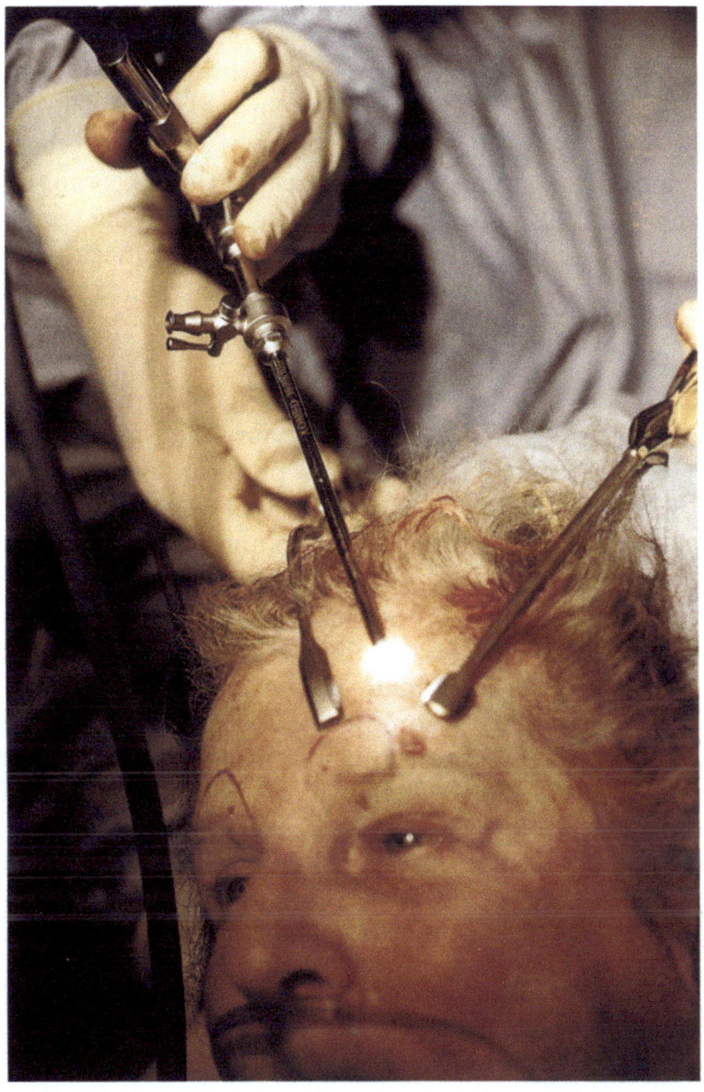

FIGURE 4.1. Endoscope with dissecting instruments. Note forehead markings 2 cm from supraorbital notch. (Courtesy of Shoib Myint, D.O.)

geon creates small incisions, then places the endoscope below the skin through the incisions and tunnels it down to the brows. After an optical cavity has been formed, the surgeon can visualize the particular nerves, vessels, and muscles that need to be dissected. The forehead is released from connections that depress it and attach it to bone. Either temporary or permanent fixation screws are used to lift up the entire forehead and secure it in its new position. Furthermore, the muscles that cause wrinkles between the eyebrows are resected to help eliminate these rhytids.

The main advantages of the endoscopic technique are smaller incisions, which are easily hidden even in thinning hair, and quicker recovery time than in the traditional coronal approach. Endoscopic techniques may also reduce the incidence of skin numbness and possible hair loss after surgery in comparison to the coronal approach. Furthermore, in men with frontal balding, endoscopic techniques can help to create a smaller scar, which is easier to conceal. Attention to several important steps in the procedure can help to reduce the occurrence of complications.

Procedure

Creation of the optical cavity in the forehead usually proceeds in the subperiosteal plane. Because this plane is avascular, dissection can be performed rapidly and safely without endoscopic visualization. The surgeon can initially develop this plane for 2 to 3 cm in the posterior direction, maintaining a "rough" feel of the periosteal elevator on bone. Once the correct plane has been confirmed, dissection can proceed anteriorly. If the correct plane is not initially entered, the periosteum may become shredded at the wound edge. The surgeon should preserve the periosteum around the anterior wound because this tissue will later be placed under tension during fixation.

Dissection in the subperiosteal plane can be performed without endoscopic visualization throughout most of the forehead (Fig. 4.2). Elevation can proceed laterally to the conjoint tendon, and anteriorly to the brow and base of the nose. Visualization with the endoscope should be performed when dissecting within 2 cm of the supraorbital notch.

Identifying and maintaining the correct plane in the temporal region is of critical importance. The surgeon must remember that under the skin and subcutaneous tissue is the *superficial temporal fascia, which contains the frontal (temporal) branch of the facial nerve,* along with the temporal artery and vein. This is a thin fascial layer, which rests superior to the deep temporal fascia.

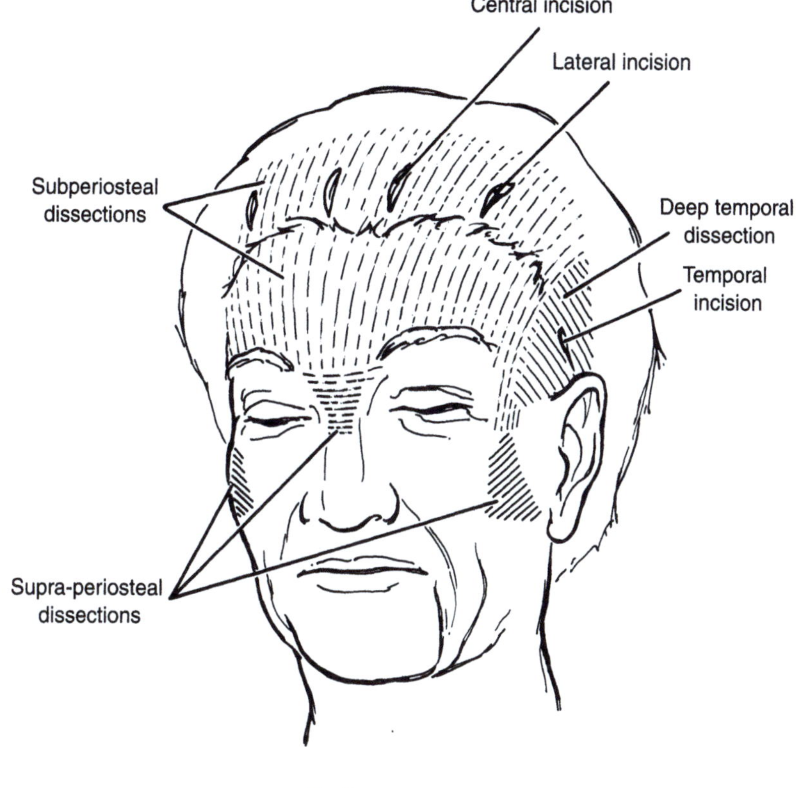

FIGURE 4.2. Recommended planes of dissection and incisions for endoscopic browlift. (Reproduced with permission from Endoscopic forehead lift. In: Nesi FA, Gladstone GJ, Brazzo BG, et al, eds. *Oph-thalmic and Facial Plastic Surgery: A Compendium of Reconstructive and Aesthetic Techniques.* Thorofare, NJ: Slack Incorporated, 2000:219–225.)

The deep temporal fascia is easily recognized as a thick, white glistening layer, firmly attached to the temporalis muscle. When attempting to identify the correct fascial layer, the surgeon should move the skin edges and observe the position of the fascia. The superficial temporal fascia will move with the skin, whereas the deep fascia remains stationary over the muscle. Upon incising the deep fascia, the surgeon can clearly visualize the dark red temporalis.

The dissection should proceed between the superficial and deep temporal fascial layers. These planes separate easily with blunt dissection. If resistance is encountered, the wrong plane may have been entered. Dissection may proceed rapidly in all directions and is safest if performed with endoscopic guidance when anterior to the hairline.

Joining the forehead and temporal cavities is necessary to mobilize the appropriate structures. After the temporal dissection has been completed, a periosteal elevator is placed through the temporal incision along the conjoint tendon and advanced against moderate resistance into the forehead cavity. Entry into the proper plane can be confirmed with endoscopic visualization through a forehead incision. Metzenbaum scissors can be used to incise the entire tendon, down to the orbital rim.

Release of the brow is performed along the superior and lateral orbital rim. Through the temporal incision, the surgeon should be careful to avoid the sentinel vein (a branch of the zygomaticotemporal vein), which rests lateral to the brow at the level of the frontozygomatic suture. This vein may be cauterized with bipolar cautery.

Dissection may be carried safely to the zygomatic arch. The *frontal branch of the facial nerve runs over the arch*, so care must be exercised near this structure. As long as dissection remains deep to the superficial temporal fascia, this nerve will not be encountered. Dissection should proceed anteriorly to the orbital rim, with release of the lateral canthal tendon.

The most tedious part of the procedure involves identification of the neurovascular bundle (Fig. 4.3) and release of the periosteum over the superomedial orbital rim (Fig. 4.4). The supraorbital nerve usually emerges from the supraorbital notch, but the entire nerve, or just a branch of it, may enter through a foramen superior to the rim. When the surgeon has identified the nerve and surrounding vessels, dissection can proceed through the periosteum.

The surgeon may choose to perform myectomy or myotomy on the depressor muscles of the brow, according to the preoperative plan.

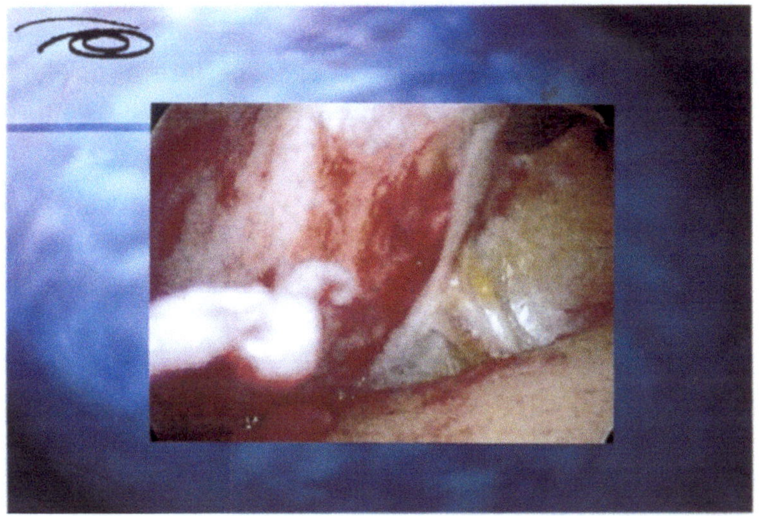

FIGURE 4.3. Identification of neurovascular bundle. (Courtesy of Shoib Myint, D.O.)

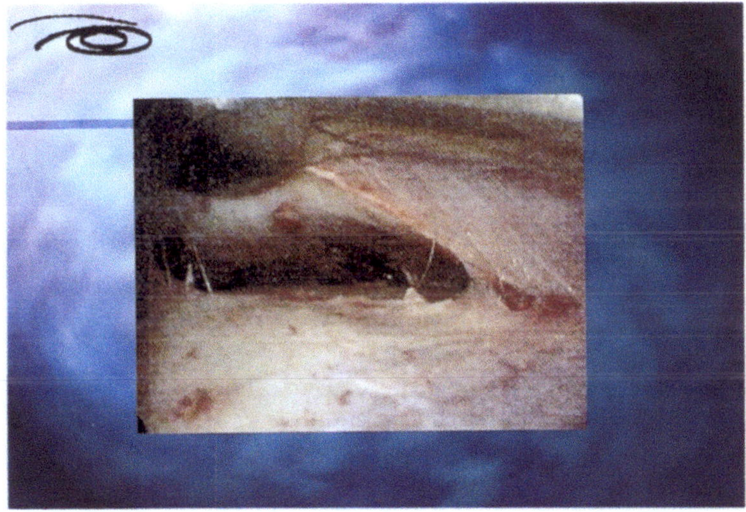

FIGURE 4.4. Complete release of periosteum over orbital rim. (Courtesy of Shoib Myint, D.O.)

Fixation of the forehead is recommended by most surgeons, although techniques vary (Fig. 4.5). The brow can be elevated by a predetermined amount, usually 1.0 to 1.5 cm. The lateral forehead incisions will usually provide the appropriate elevation and contour, and

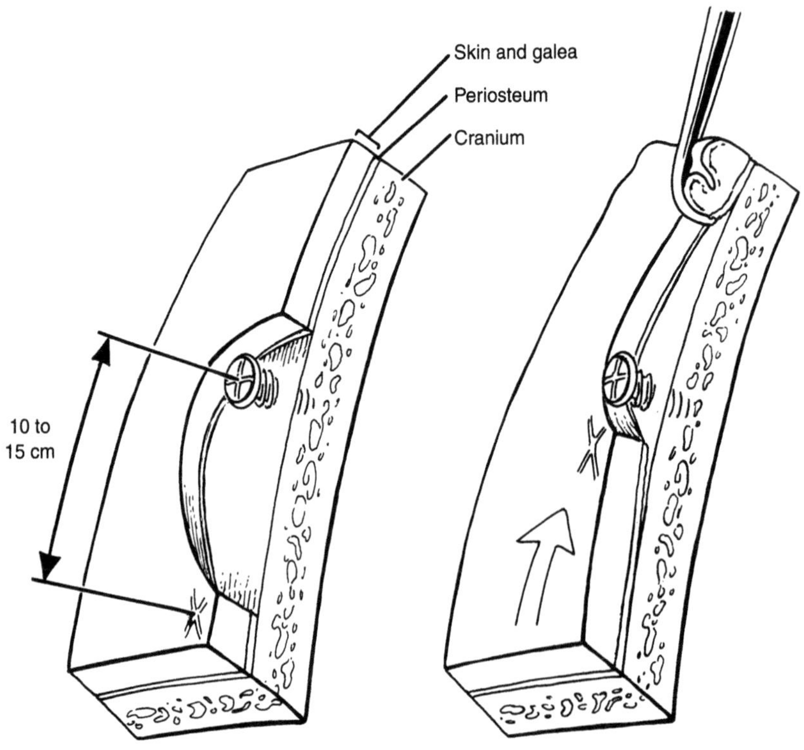

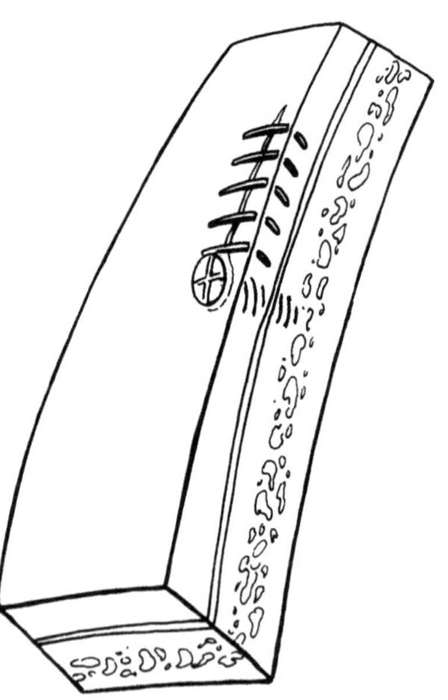

FIGURE 4.5. Elevation and fixation of the brow can be accomplished with many techniques, including screw fixation and staple closure. (A) Screw is placed into outer calvarium at a predetermined distance from anterior aspect of initial incision. (B) Sutures are placed through the periosteum; after the forehead has been elevated, the sutures are tied to the anchoring device. (C) The wound is closed. (Reproduced with permission from Endoscopic forehead lift. In: Nesi FA, Gladstone GJ, Brazzo BG, et al, eds. *Ophthalmic and Facial Plastic Surgery: A Compendium of Reconstructive and Aesthetic Techniques.* Thorofare, NJ: Slack Incorporated, 2000: 219–225.)

Forehead Lift

fixation along the midline is seldom necessary if the depressors have been weakened and the periosteum released.

Before closing the temporal incision, a small "advancement" of the superficial temporal fascia may be possible and can provide stabilization of the lateral brow. The superficial fascia anterior to the incision can be sutured to the stable deep fascia posterior to the incision with several 3-0 Vicryl sutures. Closure of all skin incisions may be accomplished with staples. However, the surgeon can obtain more accurate tissue apposition by placing several 3-0 Prolene sutures at each site. The wounds are under little tension and tend to heal with minimal scarring.

COMPLICATIONS

• David Rosenberg

Injury to the frontal (temporal) branch of the facial nerve is perhaps the most serious complication associated with brow surgery. If the correct surgical plane is maintained at all times, injury to the nerve will be very uncommon. Transection of the nerve will result in irreversible consequences. However, most instances of postsurgical nerve injury are temporary and often cause only partial paresis. In the majority of such cases, patients fully recover within 6 months.

If asymmetry is bothersome to the patient, unilateral Botox injections will provide temporary improvement. Transection of the contralateral frontal branch will provide symmetry in chronic situations, but most patients and surgeons prefer not to consider such drastic measures.

Inadequate elevation of one or both brows is the most common aesthetic problem following endoscopic browlift. Complete release of the periosteum from the orbit and forehead must be accomplished prior to fixation. If periosteal attachments remain at the time of fixation, maximal elevation will not take place at the time of surgery, and more descent will occur in the healing phase.

Some patients have brow asymmetry prior to surgery, and this observation should be demonstrated to them. Overcorrection of the low brow may be attempted during surgery, to attempt to create symmetry of the brows. However, many brows remain slightly (although less) asymmetric after surgery, while at a higher level. Patients who are aware of these points prior to surgery tend to be more satisfied postoperatively.

Excessive elevation is seldom a problem. Most brows will descend several millimeters following surgery, so that even brows that initially appear to be high will fall to an acceptable height.

Injury to the supratrochlear and supraorbital nerves will result in forehead and scalp paresthesias and anesthesia. As with damage to the frontal nerve, most such injuries are temporary and involve "bruising" the nerve rather than transection. In long-standing cases, most patients probably are no longer aware of the anesthesia and are rarely bothered by paresthesias.

Hair loss around the incision is common and often temporary. The surgeon must discuss this possibility with all patients. Some incision sites form a significant scar, and patients are bothered by localized alopecia as well as the irregular contour. Meticulous closure of the wound with sutures may give better contour and draw less attention to the incision site. Excision of a large scar or area of alopecia with primary closure is one option of reducing the appearance of an incision site.

Hematoma and seroma formation may occur in the immediate or early postoperative period. Ecchymosis and edema are common following browlift and tend to be greatest 1 or 2 days after surgery, around the brow and eyelids. Hematomas and seromas may gradually enlarge while the surrounding edema subsides. They are often discovered along the hairline or temporal region, areas that tend to demonstrate minimal edema and ecchymosis.

Treatment usually involves fluid aspiration with a needle. Repeat aspirations are commonly needed, with progressively smaller volumes removed. Even if fluid accumulation is not noticeable to the patient, aspiration should be performed to reduce the occurrence of tissue necrosis and infection.

Coronal Forehead Lift

The coronal forehead lift has for the most part been replaced by the endoscopic technique; however, it remains an effective method for lifting the upper face. An incision is made behind the hairline, extending from behind one ear, across the entire top of the head, to the other ear. The skin of the forehead is pealed down to the level of the brow and then the whole unit is pulled up, toward the top of the head, and any excess skin of the scalp is removed.

Because of the location of the resulting scar, this technique has little use in men with frontal balding, thin hair, or a receding hairline. If adequate hair is present, however, the coronal lift can be expected to produce a relatively long-lasting upper facelift with significant improvement of wrinkles of the forehead and between the eyebrows.

Midforehead, Direct, and Internal Browlift

The midforehead browlift, direct browlift, and internal browpexy are all excellent procedures for men with droopy eyebrows who are balding and do not want incisions on the scalp or in patients who wish to undergo a somewhat less extensive procedure than those just described. The three procedures differ slightly, and each works best in certain cases.

The midforehead browlift is a useful option for correcting ptotic brows in men who have forehead rhytids that can conceal the scar. In the midforehead lift, an incision is made in the middle of the forehead in an existing rhytid. The brow is lifted through this incision, secured to the underlying muscle, and the incision is meticulously closed to minimize scarring. Usually within 4 to 6 weeks the scar is adequately hidden within the wrinkle. The most common complications are scars in the forehead from direct or midforehead browlifts. These usually fade with time; however, it may take up to a year to see the final result.

The *direct browlift* is very similar to the midforehead lift except that the incision is made at the top border of the eyebrow. This procedure is more useful in men who do not have prominent forehead wrinkles to hide the midforehead incision but do have abundant brow hair to hide the direct scar.

The *internal browpexy* is performed through an incision in the crease of the eyelid below the eyebrow. The eyebrow is then lifted and reattached to the underlying bone by means of subcutaneous sutures. The advantages to the direct browlift include a well-hidden scar in the crease of the eyelid and relatively rapid recovery. However, the direct browlift cannot achieve as much elevation as either the endoscopic or coronal approaches, and the desired effect may not last as long.

REFERENCES

1. Endoscopic forehead lift. In: Nesi FA, Gladstone GJ, Brazzo BG, et al, eds. *Ophthalmic and Facial Plastic Surgery: A Compendium of Reconstructive and Aesthetic Techniques*. Thorofare, NJ: Slack Incorporated; 2000:219–215.

2. Endoscopic forehead and browlift. In: Keller GS, ed. *Endoscopic Facial Plastic Surgery*. St Louis: Mosby-Year Book; 1997:49–81.

5

ASIAN BLEPHAROPLASTY

• Steven Chen

Upper blepharoplasty is the most commonly performed aesthetic procedure among affluent Asians.[1] The vast majority of patients desire the formation of an upper lid crease, or "double eyelid." This procedure has been given various names such as "double eyelid procedure," "Oriental blepharoplasty," "lid crease procedure," and "Asian blepharoplasty." The term "Asian blepharoplasty" is preferable because this includes the various ethnic groups inhabiting the Eastern Hemisphere.

The terms "single" and "double" are used frequently by both the general public and the medical profession to describe eyelids. A single eyelid lacks a crease, which is accompanied by a fullness of the pretarsal tissues. In contrast, a double eyelid possesses a crease, which is created by a folding of the eyelid skin (Fig. 5.1). Approximately 50% of Asians have an upper lid crease, which can be complete, partial, or intermittent. Many patients requesting blepharoplasty desire the formation of a crease, or a double eyelid. Others may desire enhancement of a preexisting crease. A common misconception

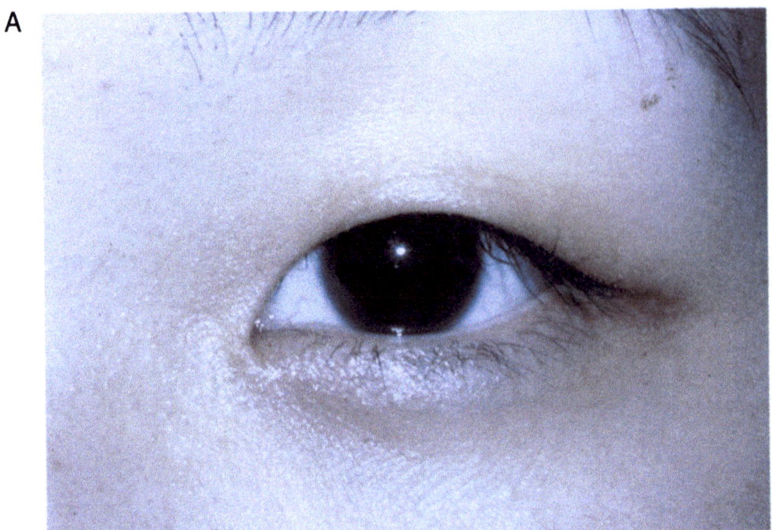

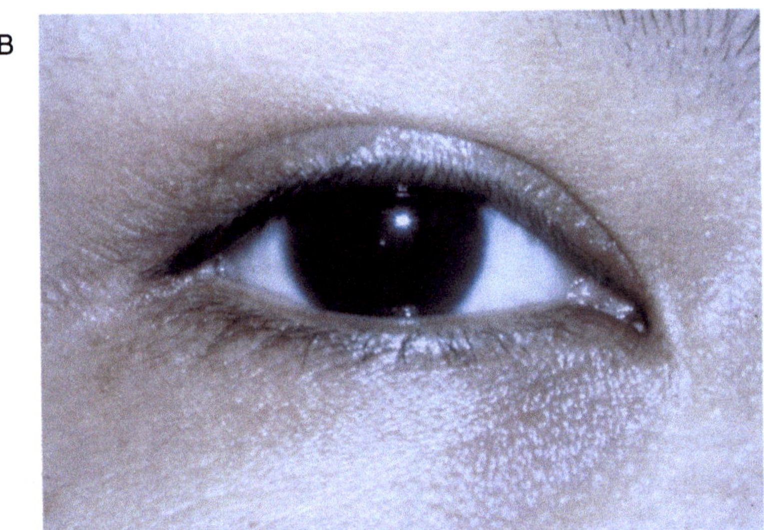

FIGURE 5.1. Asian eyelid creases: (A) "single" eyelid and (B) "double" eyelid.

is that the endpoint of Asian blepharoplasty is the creation of a more "Westernized" appearance.[2] In fact, most patients prefer an enhancement of their Asian features; they desire to have an eyelid crease like other Asians.[3] In the Asian patient, the anatomy of the upper eyelid, aesthetic goals, and surgical techniques are vastly different from that of Caucasian patients. To be proficient in Asian blepharoplasty, the surgeon must be cognizant of these differences.

ANATOMY

In what has been referred to as a classic description of Asian eyelid anatomy, Doxonas and Anderson[4] demonstrated in the upper eyelids of Caucasian and Asian patients important anatomical differences that arise from the relationship of the orbital septum to the levator aponeurosis. The levator palpebrae superioris originates from the orbital apex and courses anteriorly in the superior orbit. As it passes through the superior transverse ligament (Whitnall's ligament), the transition from levator muscle to levator aponeurosis occurs. The levator aponeurosis then fuses with the lower anterior surface of the tarsal plate. These distal aponeurotic fibers also interdigitate with the pretarsal orbicularis muscle to produce an eyelid crease.

The largest concentration of these interdigitations is along the superior tarsal border. The extent to which the levator aponeurosis interdigitates with the pretarsal orbicularis determines whether the crease will be complete, partial, or intermittent. Among Asians, approximately 50% lack these interdigitations, which are responsible for the crease.

In Caucasians the orbital septum fuses to the levator aponeurosis above the superior tarsal border. The intact septum prevents the anterior prolapse of orbital fat. In Asians, however, the orbital septum fuses with the levator aponeurosis well below the superior tarsal border (Fig. 5.2). This lower insertion results in two important differences from the Caucasian eyelid. First, the preaponeurotic fat pad extends more anteriorly and inferiorly, giving the upper eyelid a "fuller" appearance and making the crease, if present, less discernible. Second, the inferior extension of the orbital septum may prevent the terminal fibers of the levator aponeurosis from forming interdigitations with the pretarsal orbicularis muscle. As a result, the upper eyelid crease in Asians may be absent or poorly developed.[5]

More recently, some investigators have challenged this classic description of Asian eyelid anatomy.[6,7] These authors report a higher septal insertion point than previously believed. They report that the preaponeurotic fat sags anteriorly and inferiorly in front of the tarsus, bound anteriorly by a loose, movable orbital septum.

The presence of fibroadipose layer between the orbicularis muscle and the orbital septum also may also contribute to the presence or absence of an eyelid crease. This layer, which has been termed submuscular fibroadipose tissue, appears to be more prominent in Asians than in Caucasians. This layer may interfere with eyelid crease formation and may contribute to the characteristic convexity of the Asian upper eyelid.

These varying reports are consistent with the variable crease formation observed in Asian patients. Some patients have high arching upper eyelid creases with a somewhat Westernized appearance, while others have a lower more classically Asian appearance. Furthermore, some have a partial or intermittent crease, while others demonstrate no crease whatsoever. Because of these variations, the surgeon cannot take a single-minded, rigid approach to the Asian patient. The surgeon must measure the crease height, if present, and also take into account the redundancy of upper eyelid skin. In general, Asian blepharoplasty is less concerned with debulking of the upper eyelid tissues than with formation or enhancement of an eyelid crease. Skin excision may be warranted in older patients but is generally less than with Caucasian patients of similar age. In younger patients, little or no skin should be excised.

The height of the crease differs significantly among Caucasians and Asians, notably owing to the differences in the height of the tarsal plate. The tarsal height is 10 to 12 mm in Caucasians compared with 6 to 8 mm in Asians. As a result, the Asian crease is somewhat lower. One must be careful when interpreting a patient's desire to look more "Western." Surgeons who attempt to create a Western crease on an

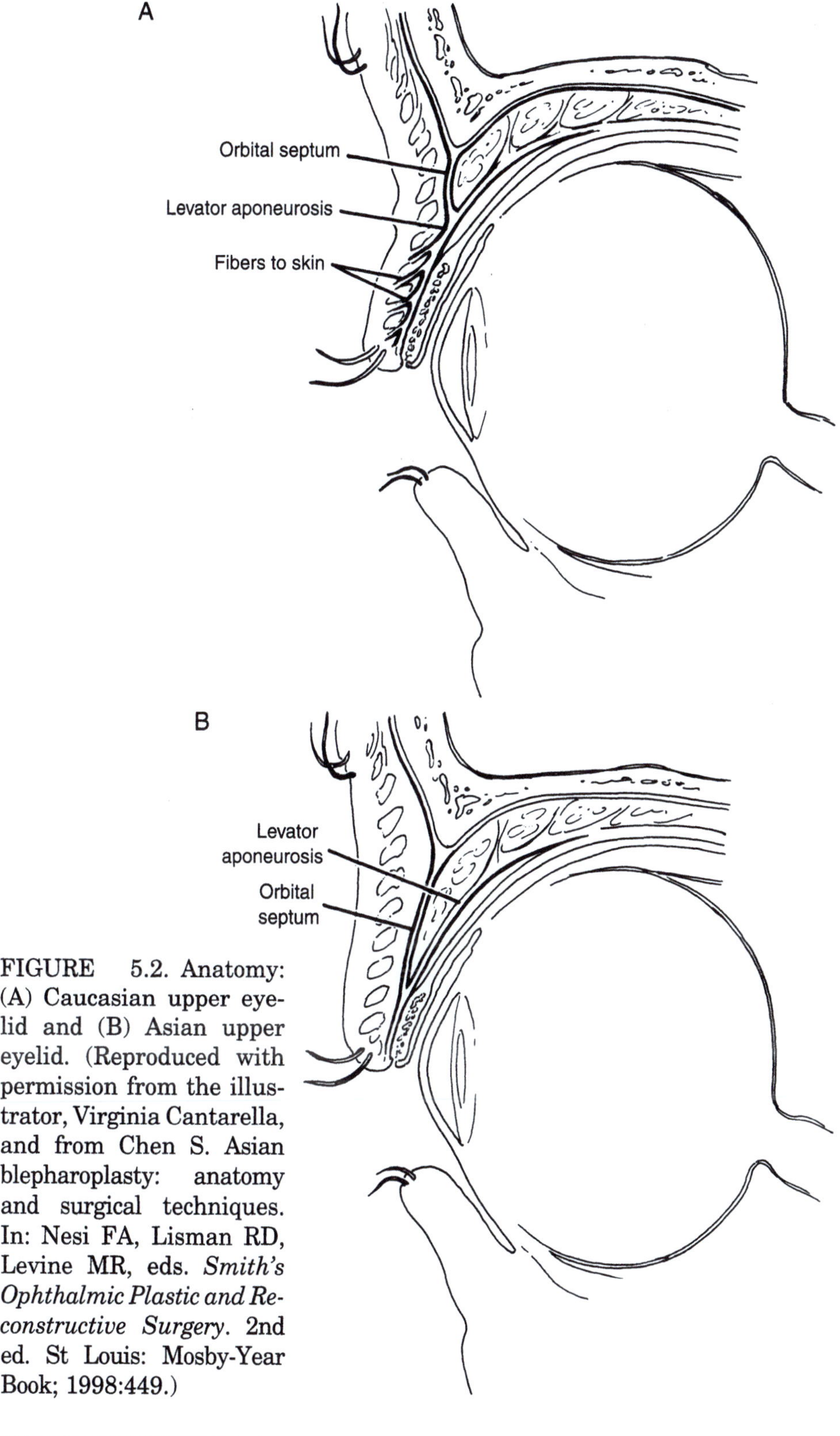

FIGURE 5.2. Anatomy: (A) Caucasian upper eyelid and (B) Asian upper eyelid. (Reproduced with permission from the illustrator, Virginia Cantarella, and from Chen S. Asian blepharoplasty: anatomy and surgical techniques. In: Nesi FA, Lisman RD, Levine MR, eds. *Smith's Ophthalmic Plastic and Reconstructive Surgery*. 2nd ed. St Louis: Mosby-Year Book; 1998:449.)

Asian patient may produce an unusually high eyelid crease, resulting in an unnatural appearance; the majority of patients will be unhappy with this result.

In the lower eyelid, the anatomical differences are subtler owing to the lack of a lid crease in both Caucasians and Asians. In Asians, the orbital septum fuses with the lower lid retractors in a slightly higher position than with Caucasians. This allows the preaponeurotic fat to prolapse forward, producing a fuller lid. In addition, the higher septal insertion may block the subcutaneous insertion of the distal fibers of the lower lid retractors. In some cases, this blockage may allow the lower eyelid skin to override the lashes, producing an epiblepharon with secondary trichiasis.

The epicanthal fold in Asians represents a unique set of challenges. Removing epicanthal folds requires a complex series of Z- and Y-plasties. Additionally, epicanthal skin is thicker and has a higher propensity toward scarring and keloid formation. In the author's opinion, most patients do not desire elimination of the epicanthal fold, and it is best left alone in Asian patients. Rather than eliminate the epicanthal fold, the author often attempts to create a crease that tapers or blends into the epicanthal fold.

EVALUATION

As with any type of aesthetic procedure, the surgeon should determine what the patient hopes to achieve. There must be clear communication between the surgeon and the patient regarding the shape and height of the crease desired. Patients seeking cosmetic surgery often have not thought clearly about how they wish their eyelids to appear and consequently do not know exactly what they want. For discussion purposes, it is helpful to have the patient bring pictures of Asian models in fashion magazines and old photographs of themselves. These visual aids help the surgeon to discover the patient's concept of beauty and to determine whether the desired results are obtainable.

It must be made clear what surgery realistically can achieve. A patient may have unrealistic expectations about what surgery can accomplish: promotion in a career, improvement of a relationship, and so on. Common misconceptions must be addressed. Some patients expect no bruising or swelling, and others expect no incision and no sutures.[2] It may be helpful to have a spouse or other family member present to aid in preoperative counseling, especially if language barriers exist between the surgeon and the patient. Terms such as "double eyelid" may be more familiar to the Asian patient than "lid crease."

As with any surgical procedure, a comprehensive ophthalmic examination is mandatory prior to surgery. It is important to document preexisting ocular pathology such as dry eye and eyelid malpositions such as entropion, ectropion, and eyelid retraction. A basic secretor test should be performed on all patients to determine basal tear production. In addition, lid height, brow height and levator function should be measured. If blepharoptosis is present, its etiology must be determined and then managed appropriately. This may require simultaneous surgery on the levator aponeurosis at the time of blepharoplasty.[8,9]

Symmetry is the most important goal in eyelid surgery because when people make eye contact, they can detect eyelid asymmetry immediately. Therefore, any preexisting asymmetry should be documented and explained to the patient. Photographic documentation is important to demonstrate preoperative findings and to allow appreciation of improvement following surgery.

Two important measurements must be taken during the preoperative evaluation: height of eyelid crease (margin–crease distance, or MCD), if present, and height of eyelid fold (margin–fold distance, or MFD). In the author's experience, patients are often more concerned with the MFD, since it is the measurement most visibly affected by eyelid surgery and formation of the eyelid crease. Even with minimal or no skin excision, the MFD can be affected by the simple creation of the eyelid crease.

TECHNIQUES

Numerous surgical techniques have been devised to create a double eyelid. These procedures fall into one of two broad categories: suture techniques and external incision. Suture techniques involve the use of full-thickness sutures to create a scar tract between the skin and conjunctiva at the desired height, thus creating an eyelid crease.

Mikamo published the first description of the suture technique in 1896.[10] Numerous variations of the suture technique have been described,[11–13] all with one common goal: creating adhesions along the superior tarsal border between the levator aponeurosis and the overlying skin and orbicularis muscle. Various types of suture material have been advocated, some absorbable and some permanent. Suture techniques have the advantage of being relatively less invasive, and they are generally easier to perform.

However, there are relative disadvantages associated with this technique. Over time, the crease has a greater tendency to fade or disappear. Because the suture techniques do not require a large skin incision, they are contraindicated in patients requiring skin or fat removal.

The earliest description of an external incision approach dates to 1929, when Maruo published both his suturing and incision techniques.[14] The surgical approach is technically more difficult and time-consuming but, when performed properly, yields superior results. The crease is more likely to be permanent, and excess upper lid skin, herniated orbital fat, and submuscular fibroadipose tissue can be debulked if necessary.

Formation of an eyelid crease by using an external skin incision produces a crease that is more physiological or "dynamic" in appearance. This dynamic effect is achieved by fixating the superior and inferior edges of the skin incision to the levator aponeurosis, approximately at the height of the superior tarsal border. The slight redundancy of skin superiorly is allowed to drape over the incision, producing the fold or "double eyelid." The eyelid crease will be most visible when the eyes are open and will tend to disappear during downgaze or eyelid closure.[15] In contrast, suture techniques produce a "static" crease, which tends to remain visible even with eyelid closure.

Suture Techniques

After the eyelid has been anesthetized with local anesthetic, the lid is everted and the superior tarsal border identified. Three double-armed sutures are passed from the conjunctival side toward the skin surface. The sutures then can be brought out onto the skin surface and tied, or buried beneath small stab incisions.

An alternate method employs a threaded needle that may be passed through the pretarsal tissues along the superior tarsal border through several stab incisions. A 4-0 silk suture is then passed in a continuous fashion along the defect. A section of rubber catheter is sutured externally, and the compressive effect of the catheter combined with the scarring from the needle tract produce an eyelid crease.[16] In these techniques, the sutures are left in place for as little as 2 to 3 days or as long as 8 to 10 days, depending on the technique and the surgeon's assessment of postoperative crease formation.

Incisional Techniques

To determine the height of the crease, the lid is everted and the height of the tarsus is measured. The incision is then outlined, with a tapering toward the epicanthal fold, if present. The surgeon may use the same local anesthetic mixture that is used for other types of blepharoplasty. The author prefers 2% lidocaine mixed with an equal volume of 0.5% bupivicaine, both with epinephrine (1:100,000). Intravenous sedation may be used, depending on the cooperation of the patient.

Younger patients generally require little or no skin excision, whereas older patients may require greater skin removal. If the patient has a preexisting lid crease that is obscured by upper eyelid skin redundancy, a small amount of skin excision is warranted (Fig. 5.3). Again, the amount of skin excision is considerably less than with Caucasians. Alternatively, if the patient desires formation of a lid crease where none had existed, little or no skin excision is required. If any skin is excised, the amount is usually less than in patients with preexisting lid creases.

After excision of skin and orbicularis muscle, the orbital septum can be opened and the preaponeurotic fat debulked, if desired. Often, the author uses an Ellman radiosurgery unit in the partially filtered and rectified mode (cutting/coagulation) to "sculpt" the preaponeurotic fat in lieu of debulking it. The amount of fat removal required in an Asian patient is generally less than in a Caucasian. A thorough knowledge of eyelid anatomy is important. Iatrogenic damage to the levator aponeurosis, which lies beneath the orbital septum and fat, can result in ptosis and is difficult to repair. As with any form of aesthetic surgery, meticulous hemostasis must be maintained to avoid the dreaded complication of retrobulbar hemorrhage.

The most important consideration for eyelid crease formation is adherence of pretarsal skin to the anterior tarsal surface, especially at the superior tarsal border. Therefore, the surgeon should ensure that any excess submuscular fibroadipose tissue as well as preaponeurotic fat is cleared from the pretarsal location. In addition, a small strip of orbicularis muscle should be excised from the inferior skin edge to further ensure adherence of the pretarsal skin to the anterior tarsal surface. It is important to note that this debulking may be unnecessary if the patient is noted to have good eyelid crease formation at the preoperative evaluation.

The lid crease then can be formed by one of several methods. Five or six interrupted sutures incorporating skin, levator aponeurosis, and skin in each bite may be used to form the lid crease.[17] Alternatively, these sutures may incorporate skin, tarsus, and skin with each

                                    Asian Blepharoplasty

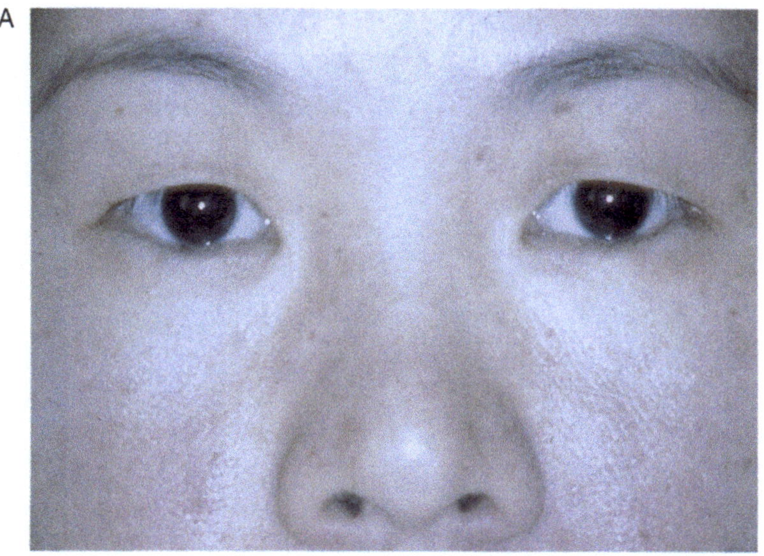

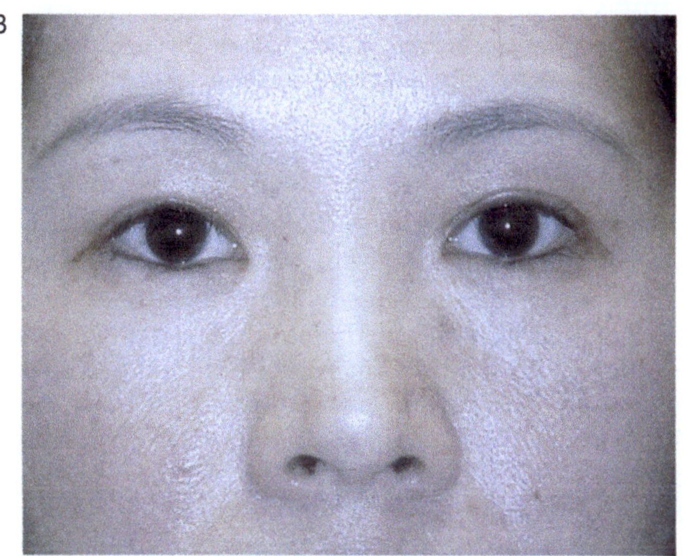

FIGURE 5.3. Asian blepharoplasty: (A) preoperative view and (B) postoperative view, with crease formed.

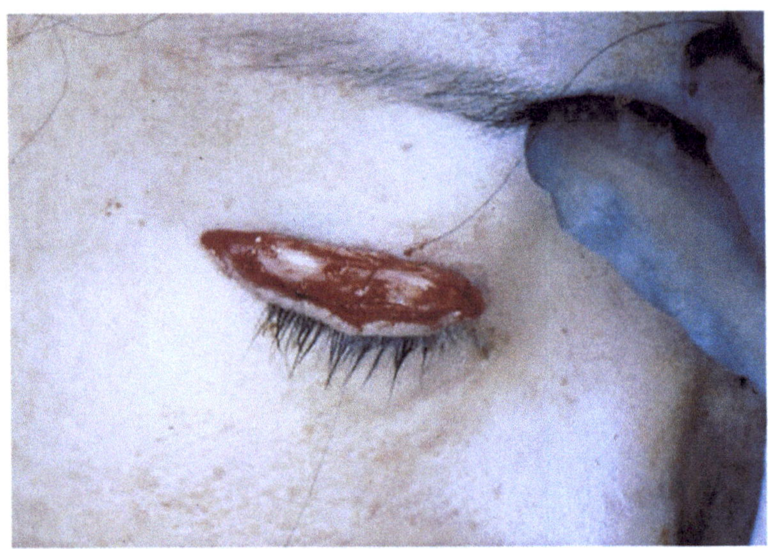

FIGURE 5.4. Intraoperative view of Asian blepharoplasty. Note placement of crease suture, which passes through the inferior skin edge, supratarsal tissue, and superior skin edge.

bite (Fig. 5.4).[18] A third method employs buried sutures incorporating tarsus and subcutaneous tissue with each bite.[19–22] Again, the key is fixation of the inferior edge of the skin incision to the superior tarsal border. The remainder of the skin incisions can be closed with either running or interrupted sutures. Permanent or absorbable sutures may be used. The author prefers interrupted sutures consisting of 6-0 silk for crease formation, combined with a running 6-0 nylon for skin closure.

If nonabsorbing sutures are used, they may be removed approximately 5 to 7 days after surgery. If a carbon dioxide laser was used to create the incisions, wound healing may be delayed and the sutures may need to remain longer. In addition, interrupted sutures used to form the eyelid crease may be left longer if crease formation appears to be delayed. The patient should expect a moderate amount of edema and ecchymosis. It is normal for the crease to appear somewhat high initially owing to postoperative edema. As the edema resolves, the crease will appear lower.

COMPLICATIONS

Numerous complications may be associated with blepharoplasty of any type. They can include common problems such as excessive or insufficient skin or fat removal, abnormalities of the lid crease, ptosis, lagophthalmos, lid retraction, exposure keratopathy, and lacrimal gland prolapse (see Chapters 1, 6, 7, and 8). Unrecognized brow ptosis (see Chapter 4) may become more apparent following blepharoplasty (especially if performed for functional reasons), as the patient's brow begins to relax. If brow asymmetry is not addressed, it is likely to affect the lid appearance, especially the margin–fold distance measurement. The patient will therefore perceive one eyelid fold to be higher than the other. Rare but serious problems such as infection, orbital hemorrhage, and blindness also may occur.[23,24]

The problems most commonly seen in Asian blepharoplasty patients are related to the height, shape, and permanence of the eyelid crease. An abnormality of the crease height most often results from excessively high placement of the crease. This situation usually occurs when one is attempting to create a more Westernized appearance, but the result is harsh and unnatural. The surgeon must always remember the anatomical differences associated with the Asian eyelid, bearing in mind that the eyelid crease will initially appear high owing to edema but will decrease in height as swelling subsides. Therefore, a patient should be advised to wait until all swelling has resolved before assessing final crease height and any need for revision. Once all swelling has resolved, the surgeon must repeat all preoperative measurements such as the MFD, MCD, and lid height.

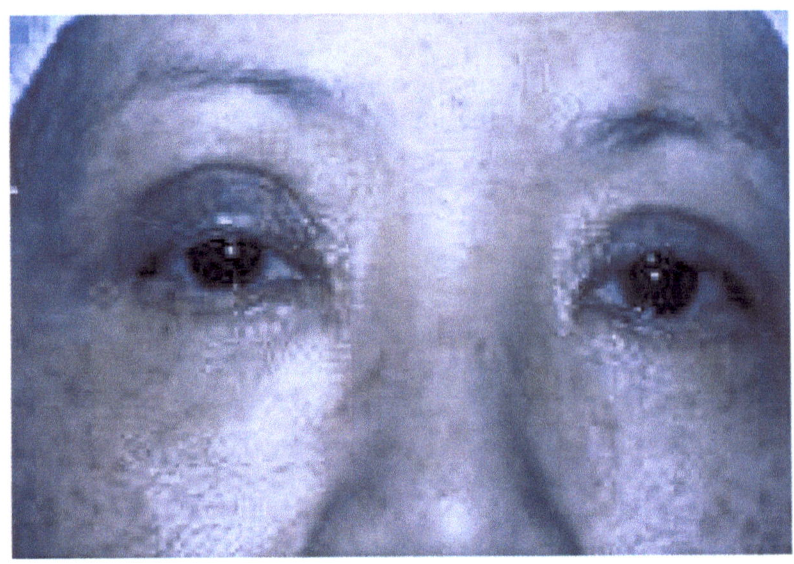

FIGURE 5.5. Iatrogenic ptosis. This middle-aged Asian woman had a blepharoplasty performed approximately 10 years prior. Subsequently, she underwent repeat blepharoplasty and later developed an iatrogenic ptosis of the right upper lid. Also note the high arch and harsh crease.

An excessively high created crease (Fig. 5.5) can be an especially vexing problem for the surgeon. It is much easier to raise the height of a crease than to lower it. Prior to attempting to lowering a crease, the surgeon must determine the height of the new crease by everting the eyelid and measuring the height of the tarsal plate. The height of the contralateral crease should also be measured. Once these measurements have been determined, an incision is made through the high lid crease. Removing a small strip of orbicularis at the inferior skin edge and debulking any submuscular fat (if present) is important prior to placement of new lid crease sutures. Again, the goal is fixation of the skin at the level of the lid crease, with free mobility of the skin superior to this. The greatest difficulty lies in preventing readherence of skin superior to the new lid crease, with re-formation of the old lid crease. Although there are no "tried and true" remedies for this problem, the author suggests that small amounts of autologous fat, or cadaveric materials such as Tutoplast (pericardium) or Alloderm (dermis) be implanted subdermally, superior to the new lid crease, in an attempt to prevent re-formation of the old crease.

Asymmetric skin removal may alter the margin–fold distance, giving the illusion that the crease is higher on one side than on the other. To achieve symmetry, the surgeon must consider removal of additional eyelid skin on the contralateral eyelid, or skin grafting to the side with excessive skin removal. It is much simpler to excise additional skin from the contralateral eyelid than to attempt skin grafting to the side with excessive removal. A skin graft would be placed above the superior tarsal border or along the superior edge of the lid crease incision.

Eyelid skin in this location is very dynamic; it folds over when the eyes are open and lies flat when they are closed. It is very difficult to prevent excessive adherence of the skin graft to the recipient bed. This situation may produce undesirable folding of the eyelid, especially if there has been excessive debulking of the underlying preaponeurotic and submuscular fat. Because the attainment of symmetry is the most important consideration, additional removal of eyelid skin from the contralateral side is often the best compromise. The surgeon and the patient should have a thorough discussion of these options prior to any revisions.

An overzealous removal of the preaponeurotic or submuscular fat pads with a secondary superior sulcus "hollowing" can further accentuate the crease height. As described earlier, many (but not all) Asians have a characteristic convexity or fullness of the upper eyelid that should not be completely eliminated. Superior sulcus deficits can be treated by autologous fat transplantation or by using acellular human dermis grafts in a manner similar to that used for patients with anophthalmic sockets. Again, because of the importance of achieving symmetry, consideration must be given to debulking fat from the contralateral side.

The surgeon should consider the possibility of an undetected ptosis when the crease of one eyelid appears higher than the other. Careful measurement of the margin reflex distance is important in the preoperative evaluation. Iatrogenic ptosis resulting from damage to the underlying levator aponeurosis requires prompt identification and repair of the levator.

If the pretarsal skin is not well connected to the underlying tarsus, especially at the superior tarsal border, all or part of the crease may disappear. This often occurs when there has been inadequate debulking of the pretarsal tissues and/or insufficient suture fixation of the inferior skin edge to the underlying pretarsal surface. The resulting appearance is a crease that is shallow, discontinuous, or obliterated. Repair requires additional debulking and replacement of lid crease sutures in the areas with inadequate crease formation. The surgeon also may consider leaving the lid crease sutures in the incision for an additional 5 to 7 days.

Multiple creases may arise after unpredictable scar formation from reoperations. Usually, the author advises a period of massaging and application of vitamin E ointment to the area, which often softens the eyelid skin and makes the folds less obvious. Occasionally, a patient will desire reversal of the lid crease procedure.[2]

Blepharoplasty in the Asian patient represents a unique set of challenges. The eyelid anatomy, aesthetic goals, and surgical techniques are vastly different from those of Caucasian patients. A common mistake made by surgeons is to apply Western concepts of anatomy, aesthetics, and surgical techniques to Asian patients. Surgeons must also be aware of the variability among Asians of the upper eyelid anatomy. The surgeon's approach must account for the presence or absence of an eyelid crease. In Caucasians, upper blepharoplasty is largely a procedure for debulking skin and preaponeurotic fat. In Asians, the primary goal is to create or enhance an eyelid crease. Debulking of skin and preaponeurotic fat is secondary and is performed mainly to enhance the appearance of the crease. Surgeons who have gained familiarity with the anatomy and surgical techniques involved will be able to help the patient achieve the desired outcome.

REFERENCES

1. Khoo BC. Some aspects of plastic (cosmetic) surgery in orientals. *Br J Plast Surg* 1969;22:60–69.

2. Chen WPD. *Asian Blepharoplasty*. Philadelphia: Butterworth-Heinemann; 1995.

3. Chen WPD. Upper blepharoplasty in the Asian patient. In: Putterman AM, ed. *Cosmetic Oculoplastic Surgery*. 2nd ed. Philadelphia: Saunders; 1993.

4. Doxonas MT, Anderson RL. Oriental eyelids: anatomic studies. *Arch Ophthalmol* 1984;102:1232–1235.

5. Amrith S. Oriental eyelids—anatomical and surgical considerations. *Singapore Med J* 1991;32:316–318.

6. Aguilar GL, Choo PH, Carter SR et al. Blepharoplasty and blepharoptosis surgery in Asians. In: Mauriello JA Jr., ed. *Unfavorable Results of Eyelid and Lacrimal Surgery: Prevention and Management*. Philadelphia: Butterworth-Heinemann; 1999:55–71.

7. Lee JS, Park WJ, Shin MS, Song C. Simplified anatomic method of double eyelid operation: septodermal fixation technique. *Plast Reconstr Surg* 1997;100:170.

   Asian Blepharoplasty

8. Jelks GW, Jelks EB. Preoperative evaluation of the blepharoplasty patient. Bypassing the pitfalls. *Clin Plast Surg* 1993;20(2):213–223.

9. Stasior OG, Ballitch HA. Ptosis repair in aesthetic blepharoplasty. *Clin Plast Surg* 20(2):247–253;269–273.

10. Mikamo K. A technique in the double eyelid operation. *J Chugaishinpo* 1896.

11. Uchida K. The Uchida method for the double-eyelid operation in 1,523 cases *Jpn J Ophthalmol* 1926;30:593.

12. Chashi K. The double eyelid operation using electrocautery. *Jpn Rev Clin Ophthalmol* 1951;46:723.

13. Pang HG. Surgical formation of upper lid fold. *Arch Ophthalmol* 1961;65:783–784.

14. Maruo M. Plastic construction of a "double-eyelid." *Jpn Rev Clin Ophthalmol* 1929;24:393–406.

15. Fernandez LR. Double eyelid operation in the Oriental in Hawaii. *Plast Reconstr Surg* 1960;25:257–264.

16. Yang PY. Double eyelid operation by the twisted needle and compressive suturing technique. *Chin J Plast Surg Burn* 1987;3:191–192.

17. Fernandez LR. The East Asian eyelid—open technique. *Clin Plast Surg* 1993;20(2):247–253.

18. Sayoc BT. Plastic construction of the superior palpebral fold. *Am J Ophthalmol* 1954;38:556–559.

19. Sheen JH. Supratarsal fixation in upper blepharoplasty. *Plast Reconstr Surg* 1974;54:424–431.

20. Sheen JH. A change in the technique of supratarsal fixation in upper blepharoplasty. *Plast Reconstr Surg* 1977;59:831–834.

21. Weingarten CZ. Blepharoplasty in the Oriental eye. *Trans Am Acad Ophthalmol Otolaryngol* 1976;82:442–226.

22. Putterman AM, Urist MJ. Reconstruction of the upper eyelid crease and fold. *Arch Ophthalmol* 1976;94:1941–1954.

23. Dortzbach RK, ed. *Ophthalmic Plastic Surgery: Prevention and Managment of Complications*. New York: Raven Press; 1994.

24. Lowry JC, Bartley GB. Complications of blepharoplasty. *Survey Ophthalmol* 1994;38(4):327–335.

References   *73*

PART II

PTOSIS

6

EXTERNAL LEVATOR ADVANCEMENT

• César A. Sierra
• Frank A. Nesi

A spectrum of conditions affects the upper eyelid height, but the most common is acquired ptosis secondary to aponeurosis disinsertion. The successful outcome of ptosis repair depends on the preoperative history, evaluation, and formulation of the most adequate plan of management.

EVALUATION

A careful history should determine both functional and cosmetic concerns that the patient might have. "Droopy eyelid" is one of the most common complaints encountered by the surgeon. Frequently, excess and overhang of eyelid skin plays a significant part of the patient's concerns. Using a mirror when discussing the problem is extremely valuable to elicit the patient's expectations. Furthermore, this simple technique can be used at the end of the evaluation to help the physician explain the plan of management and the expected surgical outcome.

Occasionally patients do not remember the time of onset of the problem, and it is helpful to review old photographs such as a driver's license or, in cases of suspected congenital ptosis, childhood photographs. Past history of injury or previous facial, eyelid, and ocular surgery is an essential part of the evaluation. Progression of the ptosis as well as variations in eyelid height during the day should be thoroughly investigated. Detailed questions regarding bleeding tendency and the use of blood thinners including herbal supplements should be reviewed in every patient if surgical management is required.

Patients with dehiscence of the levator aponeurosis classically present with blockage of the superior visual field, good levator function, and an elevated eyelid crease height.

In addition to a complete history, the preoperative evaluation includes several eyelid measurements that are essential to make an accurate diagnosis and guide the surgical plan. The most critical of these is the levator function, or eyelid excursion. This determines the power the levator muscle has to elevate the upper eyelid. Involuntary use of the frontalis muscle is commonly observed in patients with ptosis to compensate for the superior visual blockage. The upper eyelid excursion is an accurate and reproducible measurement, provided the physician blocks the action of the forehead–eyebrow complex. The eyelid excursion is measured in millimeters from extreme downgaze to upgaze. Good levator function is considered present when it measures 10 mm or more. Less excursion should lead the surgeon to consider a different procedure, such as levator resection or frontalis fixation.

The severity of the ptosis is also important, since it will indicate the amount of advancement needed with the procedure. Although the vertical palpebral fissure measurement gives an idea of the aperture of the eyelids, it is less than ideal in the evaluation of ptosis

   External Levator Advancement

or retraction. The palpebral fissure is measured from the central upper lid margin to the lower lid margin. However, it does not take into consideration the possibility of lower eyelid retraction that could lead to errors estimating the degree of ptosis. In contrast, the upper eyelid margin-to-reflex distance (MRD1) is more accurate and reproducible because it uses a fixed point of reference (i.e., corneal light reflex) and is not dependent on changes in the lower eyelid position.

The MRD1 quantifies the degree of ptosis and illustrates the amount of advancement needed. The patient is asked to fixate in primary gaze at a Finnoff light or penlight held by the examiner. The distance between the central upper eyelid margin and the corneal light reflex is measured in millimeters while the action of the frontalis muscle is blocked with the other hand. When the ptosis is severe enough to block the corneal light reflex, the eyelid is lifted until visualized and the amount of elevation is estimated and recorded as a negative measurement.

The severity of ptosis can be quantified by comparing the MRD1 with the ideal eyelid height. In unilateral ptosis the ideal height is the level of the unaffected eyelid. If bilateral, an arbitrary measurement of 4.0 to 4.5 mm is desirable only if it does not compromise preexisting ocular surface conditions such as keratitis or a glaucoma filtering bleb. In these cases it is better to proceed conservatively and raise the eyelid just enough to improve the superior visual field.

The adequacy of the Bell's phenomenon and the degree of preexisting lagophthalmos are other preoperative measurements that may dictate how high one should consider raising the ptotic eyelid. The presence of dry eye syndrome should be excluded by performing Schirmer's test and documenting absence of punctate epithelial keratopathy.

In unilateral ptosis, it is important to assess and discuss the possibility of postoperative ptosis in the contralateral eyelid (Fig. 6.1). This can be explained by the effect of Hering's law of equal innerva-

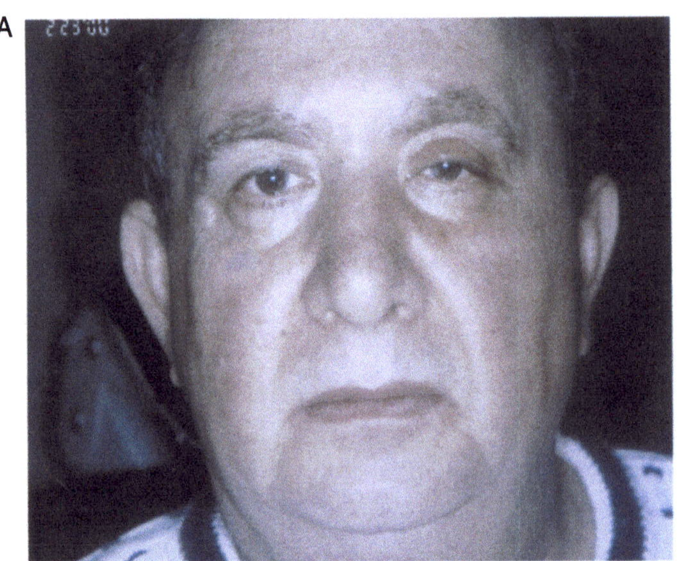

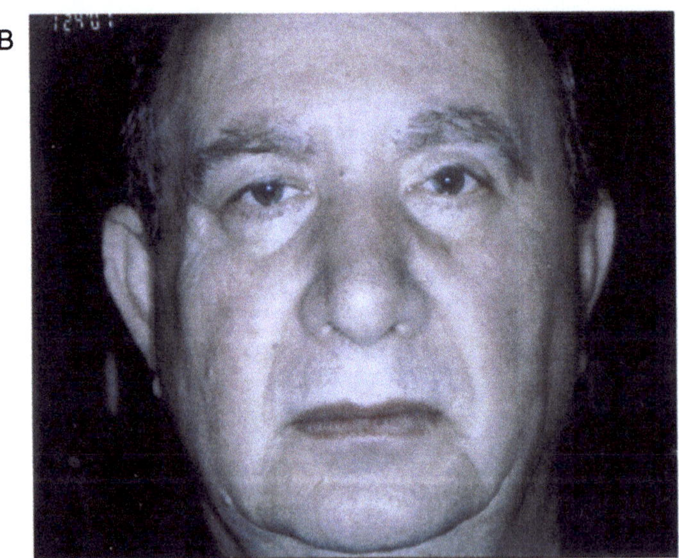

FIGURE 6.1. Hering's law. (A) Patient with left upper eyelid ptosis. (B) Following left upper eyelid ptosis repair, the level of the right upper eyelid became 1 to 2 mm lower.

                                          External Levator Advancement

tion to paired yoke muscles. After the ptotic eyelid has been corrected, less innervation is required and a weaker signal will be delivered to the "normal" side, since both levator muscles are equally innervated. The surgeon is able to evaluate this phenomenon in the office by carefully lifting the ptotic eyelid to the desired level with one finger and observing any changes this maneuver may cause on the contralateral eyelid height. In such cases, the ptosis should be repaired in stages to let the operated eyelid heal. On the second surgery, the surgeon attempts to create symmetry.

Attention should be given to the eyelid crease and fold, especially when one is considering a blepharoplasty combined with ptosis surgery. An absent or low crease may be addressed as part of a combined ptosis–blepharoplasty procedure. The eyelid margin-to-crease distance (MCD) also provides clues about the degree of the levator dehiscence. When present, the eyelid fold is gently lifted to confirm the presence and position of the crease during vertical eye movement. In non-Asian women the crease should lie 10 to 12 mm from the eyelid margin. Care should be taken to create the male crease no higher than 8 mm.

TECHNIQUE

The accuracy of ptosis repair by levator advancement depends largely on the intraoperative cooperation of the patient in opening the eyes to verify the appropriate eyelid position. Although the procedure can be performed in the office, conscious sedation should be considered for the anxious patient. Even though these patients are required to be awake during surgery, the level of comfort has improved considerably with the recent introduction of potent, short-acting intravenous anesthetics such as propofol in combination with midazolam (Versed) for induction. A starting dose of 1 mg of Versed and 40 mg of propofol in adults induces amnesia and anesthesia, facilitating the infiltration of the eyelids with local anesthetic. The advantage of propofol is its rapid half-life ($t_{1/2}$ = 2–8 min), which provides sufficient time to inject the area without causing discomfort and clears fast enough to ensure patient cooperation throughout the procedure.

The incision is marked along the eyelid crease when present and is usually made symmetric to the contralateral crease. The marking should be done with the patient in the sitting position to allow the eyelid and skin to assume their normal position. If bilateral ptosis is present and the creases are not in a desirable position, new creases should be made 8 to 10 mm from the central lid margin.

The marking is extended nasally to the area just above the upper punctum to avoid the formation of undesirable webbing or redundant skin in the medial canthal area. A noticeable scar can form at the lateral end of an incision that is extended beyond the lateral orbital rim. A fine-tipped marking pen is recommended to avoid any ambiguity at the time of skin incision.

If excess skin is present, forceps are used to determine the amount to be excised. A conservative approach is the key element of any blepharoplasty, and this "skin pinch" technique should not be employed to ascertain the maximum amount of skin that can be excised but rather to avoid removing too much skin. An aggressive approach only leads to complications such as retraction and lagophthalmos secondary to iatrogenic foreshortening of the skin and the appearance of having "short eyelids."

Instead, the surgeon must determine the smallest skin resection that will enhance the appearance of the eyelid. The area to be included in the incision should not extend below the eyelid crease inferiorly and should remain at least 10 mm from the inferior brow. The surgeon should mark the proposed skin incisions before the local anesthetic is infiltrated.

An equal volume of 2% lidocaine with epinephrine and 0.75% bupivicaine with epinephrine and hyaluronidase (Wydase) is injected subcutaneously in the previously marked area. After the patient has been prepped and draped, the incision is made along the previously marked lines with a #15 Bard–Parker blade. The incision should be deep enough to spread the skin and visualize the subcutaneous tissue. Care should be taken to avoid inadvertent damage to deeper structures. Wescott scissors are used to excise the skin and the orbicularis muscle flap. Again, the dissection should proceed in the correct plane to prevent damage to the levator complex.

Dissection of an inferior skin flap in the central portion of the eyelid exposes the anterior surface of the tarsus (Fig. 6.2). If necessary, the pretarsal orbicularis muscle is removed to expose the surface of the upper tarsus. The surgeon should be careful to avoid bleeding secondary to damage to the underlying peripheral vascular arcade

    External Levator Advancement

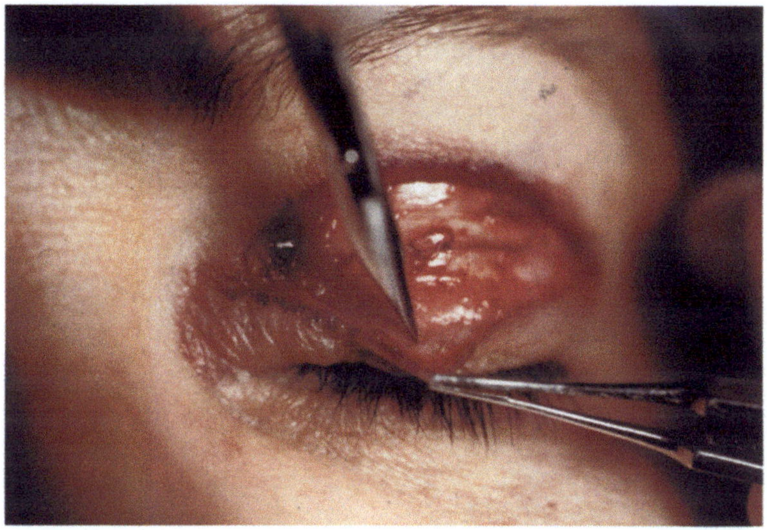

FIGURE 6.2. The tarsus must be exposed by dissecting an inferior skin flap in the central portion of the eyelid and removing pretarsal orbicularis.

and Muller's muscle. Excess bleeding will make it more difficult to gauge the correct final eyelid position. The undulating vessels of the peripheral arcade make the underlying Muller's muscle easy to identify.

The edge of the dehiscent levator aponeurosis is seen as a white line of tissue superior to the upper border of the tarsus between the orbital fat and the Muller's muscle. Toothed forceps are used to pull the edge of the levator aponeurosis inferiorly while the assistant pulls the septum anteriorly and superiorly. The entire septum is incised horizontally with high-temperature cautery.

Several points should be emphasized at this stage of the procedure to avoid accidental damage to the levator and deeper structures. First, tenting the septum 90° away from the levator aponeurosis creates a potential space between the muscle and the deeper structures. Second, the cautery (incision) should always be directed parallel to the angle of the levator aponeurosis. Third, incising the septum completely prevents its inclusion in the advanced tissues and lowers the risk of lagophthalmos (Fig. 6.3).

Once the levator complex has been adequately exposed, the eyelid is lifted off the globe. The authors prefer to pass a double-armed 6-0 silk or 5-0 Novafil suture through the central tarsus with partial thickness bites 1 to 2 mm below the superior tarsal border. A central

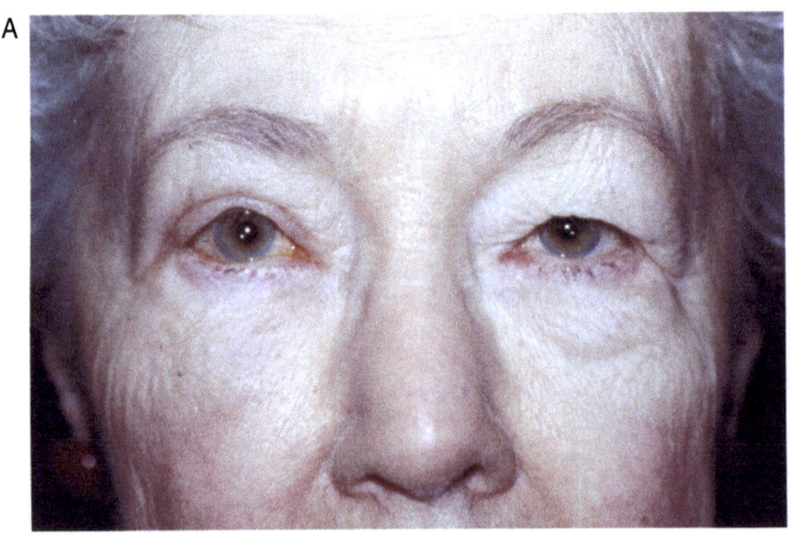

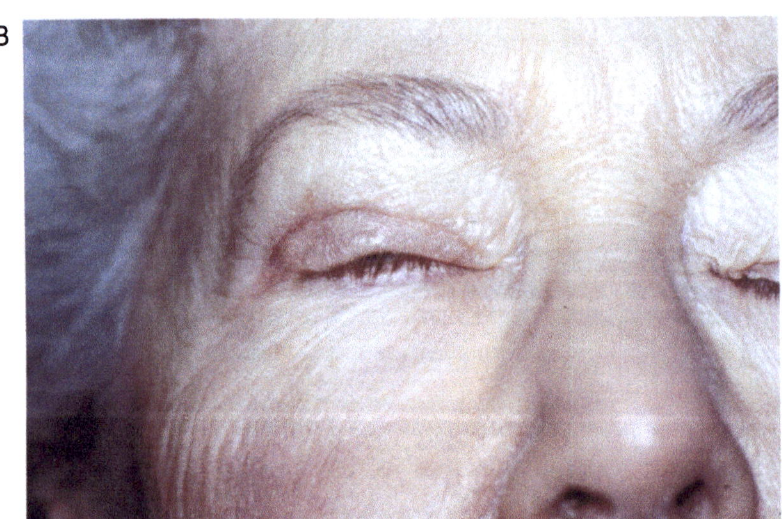

FIGURE 6.3. (A) Patient following ptosis repair of right upper eyelid. Mild central "peaking" is present. (B) Mild lagophthalmos is also present.

5 mm broad-based bite (Fig. 6.4) through the tarsus is recommended for better eyelid contour. The eyelid is always everted after each pass through the tarsus to ensure that the needle has not penetrated the full thickness of the eyelid. This maneuver will reduce the risk of suture abrasion to the globe.

Several years ago, the authors developed a new approach to levator advancement in which a single broad-based mattress suture is used rather than the traditional three-suture technique. This new procedure widens the vector of force of the central suture and eliminates the need for medial and lateral sutures, making the procedure easier to perform and resulting in better contour of the eyelid margin. The tarsal bite should be 5.0 to 5.5 mm in width.

Next, both arms of the suture are carefully passed through the levator aponeurosis in a mattress fashion, avoiding deeper tissues, such as the vascular Muller's muscle, which could lead to formation of a hematoma. The suture is tied temporarily to allow for adjustment. The patient opens both eyes and the surgeon assesses the eyelid height and contour. Frequently the patient is placed in a sitting position, which helps the patient to become more alert and the surgeon to confirm the appropriate lid height and contour. The surgeon should aim for an intraoperative overcorrection of 1 mm, since the lid tends

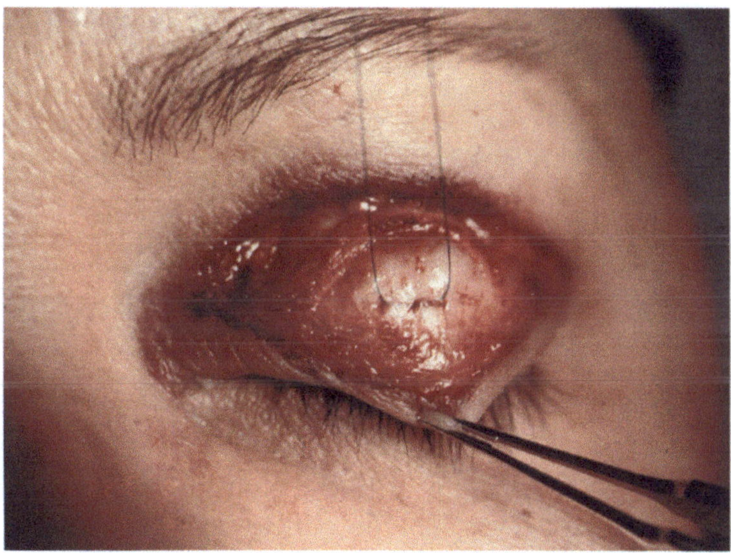

FIGURE 6.4. Placement of a single 5 mm broad-based tarsal suture. The edge of the levator muscle is seen just superior to the tarsus.

to droop this amount in the early postoperative period. Changes in the placement or tightness of the suture should be done until the correct eyelid position has been attained. The suture is tied with a permanent square knot and the lid height is evaluated once more before skin closure.

The preaponeurotic fat pads may be excised. This should be performed with the use of the "3 C's" technique: clamping the fat with a hemostat, cutting with scissors, and cauterizing with thermal and/or bipolar cautery. The stump of the fat pad is always grasped with toothed forceps before the hemostat is released, to be able to cauterize any remaining active bleeding before the fat pad retracts into the orbit.

The authors prefer a running subcuticular 6-0 Prolene suture for a seamless skin closure and painless removal. Tincture of benzoin and surgical tape are placed to protect the wound and limit disruption caused by movement of the eyelid.

The patient is instructed to apply ice packs every hour for 15 minutes during the first 48 hours. Lubrication with antibiotic ointment should be considered if postoperative lagophthalmos is an issue. The patient should avoid lifting heavy objects and bending, to reduce the risk of postoperative hemorrhage that could affect the final eyelid height or cause orbital hemorrhage if severe.

The first postoperative visit is scheduled one week after the procedure for suture removal. Eyelid height should also be assessed, and presence of lagophthalmos determined.

COMPLICATIONS

Complications from misplacement of the levator suture are most often preventable and correctable during the surgery. Placing the tarsal suture lower than the upper third of the tarsus might lead to entropion.

The width of the tarsal suture is important in obtaining proper eyelid contour. The bite should be 5.0 to 5.5 mm in width. A smaller bite may create "peaking" of the eyelid margin (Fig. 6.3A), whereas a wider tarsal bite will result in flattening of the eyelid contour. Placing the suture medial or lateral to the central 5 mm of tarsus will also inappropriately elevate the margin toward that side (Fig. 6.5). Repositioning the sutures and reassessing the eyelid contour can correct these complications.

Retraction (Fig. 6.6) results when ptosis is overcorrected, causing exacerbation of keratopathy and dry eye conditions. Lagophthalmos

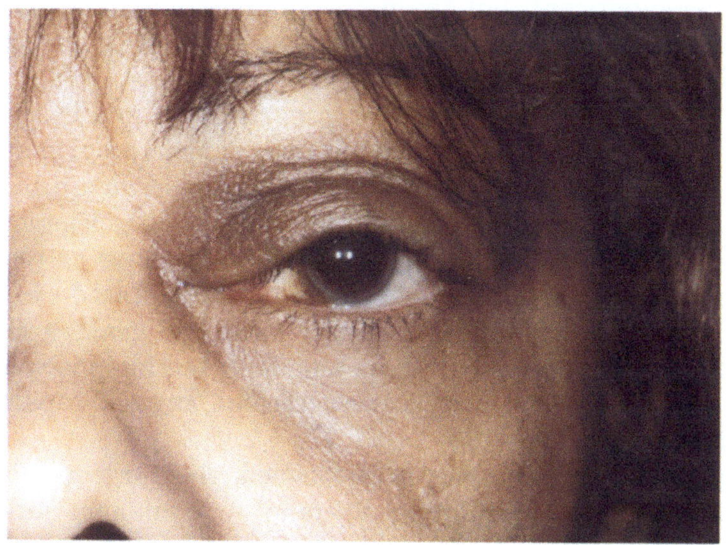

FIGURE 6.5. Following ptosis repair, this patient developed mild contour irregularity with medial ptosis.

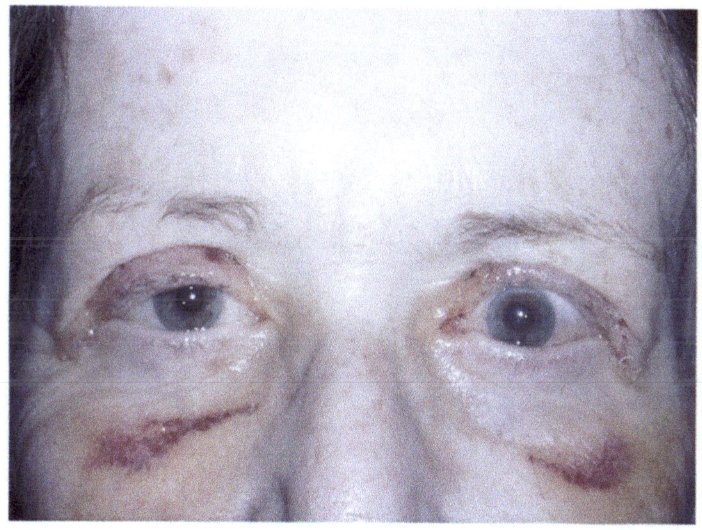

FIGURE 6.6. Mild left upper eyelid retraction, 3 days following levator advancement. The patient has eyelid asymmetry, with marked increase in keratopathy and discomfort.

may not be significant, but the patient's discomfort, and findings of corneal staining, conjunctival injection, and eyelid asymmetry point to this diagnosis.

Lagophthalmos is often noted intraoperatively and in the immediate postoperative period. This condition is seldom problematic if the surgeon had ensured that septum was not incorporated into the levator–tarsal suture (Fig. 6.7). If several millimeters of lagophthalmos persist (Fig. 6.8), the levator suture may be released or readjusted within a week of the surgery, often as an office procedure. In mild cases, the surgeon should instruct the patient to gently pull inferiorly on the eyelashes several times per day, starting one week after surgery. If this simple remedy is unsuccessful, surgical repair should be considered.

If repair of lagophthalmos is performed, the surgeon must open the initial incision and explore the wound. A permanent suture may need to be removed, and the levator may need to be recessed. Any vertical scar bands need to be identified and lysed. The surgeon pulls the eyelid inferiorly and palpates or visualizes the vertical bands

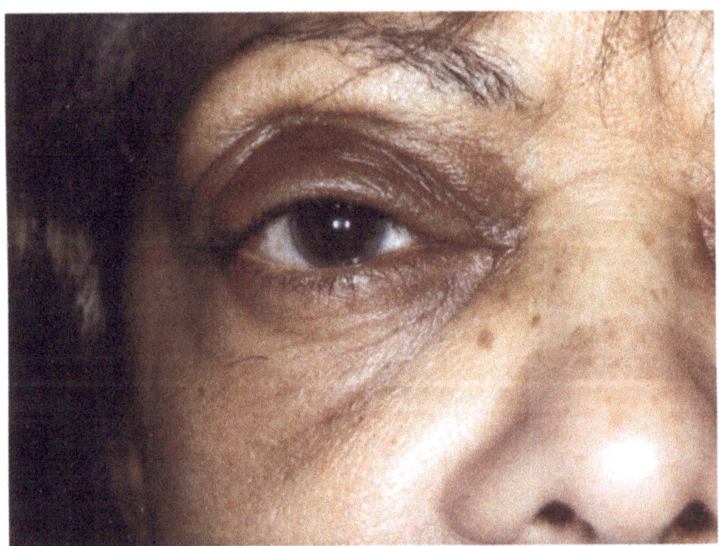

FIGURE 6.7. Following ptosis repair, this patient developed high eyelid crease with lagophthalmos, secondary to incarceration of septum.

                                    External Levator Advancement

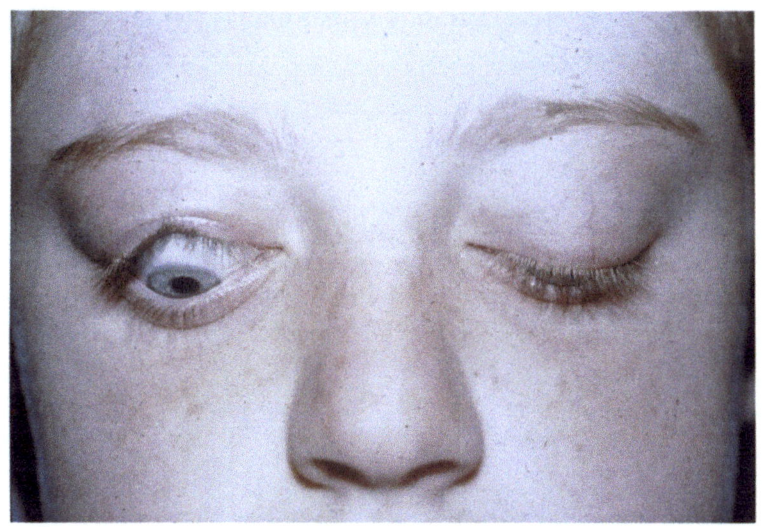

FIGURE 6.8. Severe lagophthalmos following levator advancement.

(Fig. 6.9) over the septum or levator. These bands need to be lysed. The eyelid may be secured to the cheek or lower lid for several days to prevent reoccurrence (see Chapter 12 for discussion of upper eyelid retraction repair).

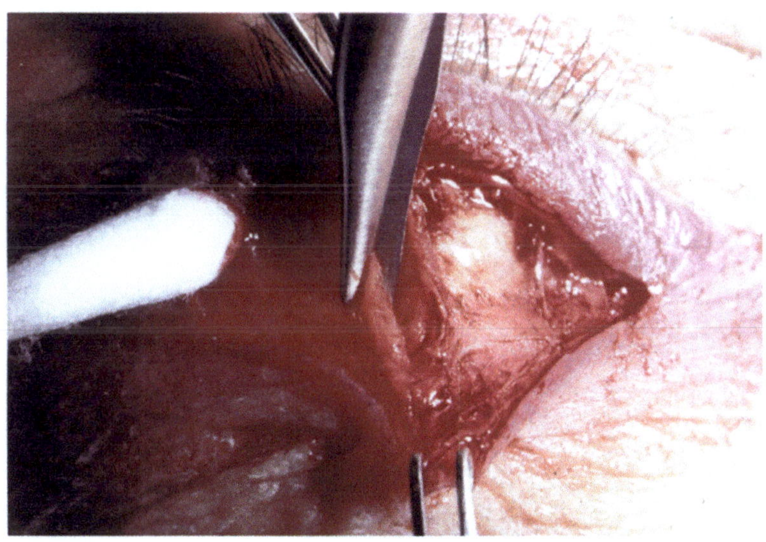

FIGURE 6.9. Vertical scar bands and attachments to septum are lysed.

Other complications common to upper eyelid surgery are discussed in Chapters 1 and 8.

REFERENCE

1. External levator advancement. In: Nesi FA, Gladstone GJ, Brazzo BG, et al, eds. *Ophthalmic and Facial Plastic Surgery: A Compendium of Reconstructive and Aesthetic Techniques.* Thorofare, NJ: Slack Incorporated; 2000:219–225.

7

MULLER'S MUSCLE–CONJUNCTIVAL RESECTION

- César A. Sierra
- Geoffrey J. Gladstone

Muller's muscle–conjunctival resection (MMCR) is reserved for patients with good levator function and mild to severe ptosis that responds adequately to phenylephrine. Excellent results have also been demonstrated in patients with minimal congenital ptosis or mild to moderate acquired ptosis, including those with Horner's syndrome and anophthalmic ptosis.

Muller's muscle is a sympathetically innervated smooth muscle that lies between the conjunctiva and the levator aponeurosis. It originates from the levator aponeurosis approximately 15 to 20 mm above its insertion on the superior tarsal border. In cases of sympathetic denervation or Horner's syndrome, the absence of adequate neurochemical input to Muller's muscle will result in mild ptosis of approximately 2.0 to 2.5 mm. Therefore, this amount of eyelid lift is attributed to Muller's muscle.

EVALUATION

The preoperative evaluation is critical because many patients with true eyelid ptosis will also present with dermatochalasis or forehead/brow ptosis and will simply describe their problem as a "droopy eyelid." A meticulous history, including previous surgeries or injuries, and a preoperative exam, should reveal clearly the type of ptosis and associated eyelid/forehead problems. It is as important to fully understand the patient's concerns and expectations as it is to determine the exact diagnosis. Before the surgery, the patient needs to understand this diagnosis, including coexistent upper lid and brow problems, as well as the plan of action and its advantages and limitations.

There are several eyelid measurements that are essential to classify the type of ptosis and guide the surgeon to the best management. Determining levator function, also called upper lid excursion, will enable the surgeon to establish the type of ptosis and to guide the surgical approach. Patients with blockage of the superior field of vision (i.e., ptosis, dermatochalasis) tend to lift the chin and use the forehead muscles to compensate for the small vertical aperture. While the examiner immobilizes the frontalis muscle with one hand on the forehead, the lid excursion is measured in millimeters from extreme downgaze to upgaze. "Good" levator function is present when this measurement is more than 10 mm.

The distance from the upper eyelid margin to corneal light reflex (MRD1) must also be established. If the eyelid lies below the pupillary light reflex, then the examiner must elevate the lid until the light is seen. This amount of elevation is estimated and recorded as a negative measurement.

Involuntary recruitment of the frontalis muscle is very common when patients with ptosis attempt to elevate the upper lids. Care must be taken to avoid underestimation of the degree of ptosis secondary to frontalis action. A simple way to elicit relaxation of these muscles is to ask the patient to look down for several seconds before returning to primary gaze. This usually prevents the patient from inadvertently raising the eyelids with the help of the forehead muscles to compensate for the ptosis. It is always a good idea to lower the intensity of the handheld light to prevent the patient from squinting, which will consequently cause underestimation of the MRD1.

The decision to perform an MMCR and the determination of the amount of conjunctiva and Muller's muscle to resect depend on the adequacy and level of response of the upper eyelid to the phenyl-

     Muller's Muscle–Conjunctival Resection

ephrine test. The MRD1 is measured before and after the instillation of topical ophthalmic phenylephrine (Fig. 7.1). Note that the lower lid retractors are the equivalent to the upper eyelid Muller's muscle and also respond to topical sympathomimetic agents, which increase the vertical height of the palpebral fissure. Unlike the palpebral fissure

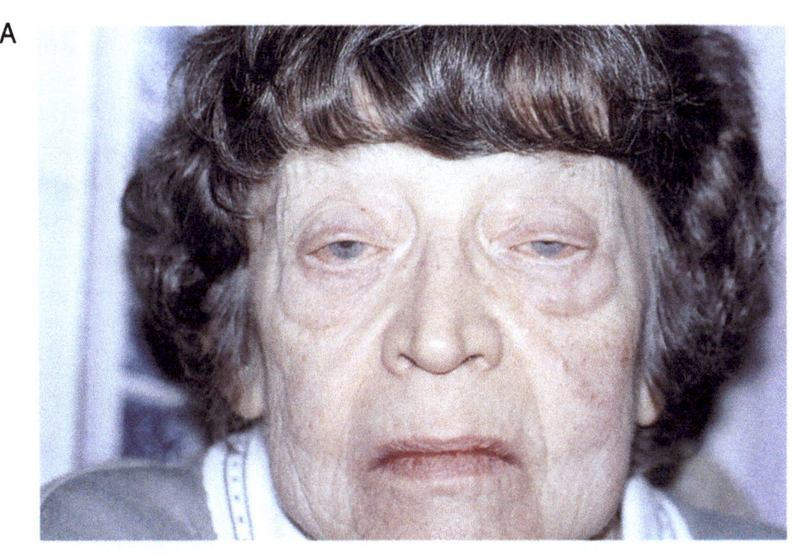

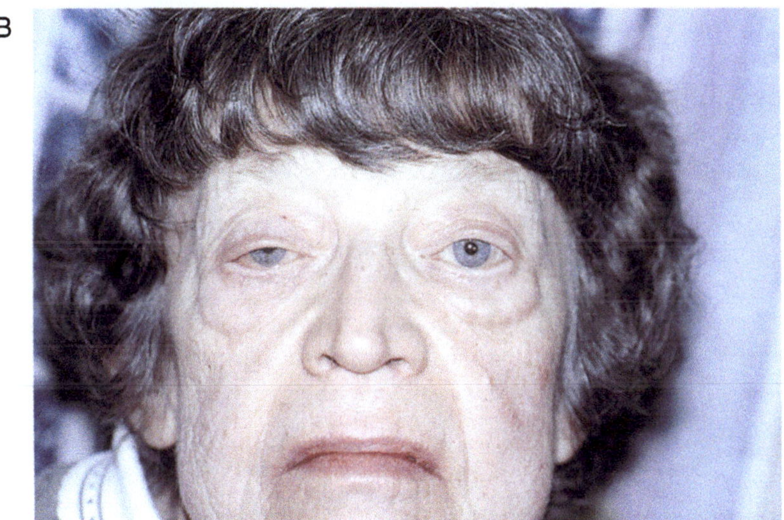

FIGURE 7.1. (A) Patient with bilateral ptosis. (B) Positive response to phenylephrine test (only left eye tested).

measurement, MRD1 is independent of the lower lid, making it more reliable and reproducible for ptosis evaluation.

Classically a concentration of 10% phenylephrine is used to stimulate this sympathetically innervated muscle. Ophthalmic tetracaine solution is given first, to avoid the burning sensation associated with phenylephrine and to prevent forceful closure of the eyelids and reflex tearing. A total of two phenylephrine drops are instilled at 5-minute intervals. Although some surgeons add a third set of drops one minute later, it does not seem to change the outcome and poses more risks of inducing side effects.

The MRD1 is measured again 3 to 5 minutes later. In unilateral ptosis, an MMCR is considered only if the "postphenylephrine" MRD1 lies within 1 mm of the normal lid height. In bilateral ptosis an arbitrary MRD1 of 4.5 mm is set as the standard and used to gauge the adequacy of the test. An 8.0 to 8.5 mm resection of conjunctiva and Muller's muscle is performed when the eyelid is elevated to a normal level after instillation of the drops. If the lid is lower but within 1 mm of the normal, more tissue is resected (8.5–9.5 mm). Conversely, less tissue is resected when the subsequent MRD1 is higher than in the normal lid (6.5–7.5 mm) (Table 7.1).

Ideally the measurements before and after phenylephrine should be made under the same light conditions. If the patient squints in response to a brighter room or Finnoff light, for example, this could potentially lead to inaccurate calculation of the amount of resection.

It should be emphasized that topical phenylephrine must be avoided in high-risk patients with known cerebral aneurysms, cerebrovascular disease, or severe coronary artery disease. The authors have found the use of 10% phenylephrine for ptosis evaluation to be safe after careful exclusion of patients with these known risk factors.

TABLE 7.1 Phenylephrine test for MMCR

Lid height post 10% phenylephrine[a]	Amount to resect (mm)
Lower	8.5–9.5
Normal	8.0–8.5
Higher	6.5–7.5

[a]Compared with the normal eyelid height in unilateral ptosis and to the standard 4.5 mm MRD1 in bilateral ptosis.

   Muller's Muscle–Conjunctival Resection

Patient selection and blockage of the puncta with a finger for 3 to 5 minutes are fundamental to avoid complications secondary to a sympathetic reaction.

Indications

MMCR is usually reserved for patients who meet all the following criteria: mild to severe ptosis, good levator function, and adequate response to the phenylephrine test.

Excellent results have been shown in patients with mild congenital ptosis, mild to moderate acquired ptosis, Horner's syndrome, and anophthalmic ptosis.

The major advantages of this posterior approach over an external approach such as levator advancement are the absence of a visible scar and the option of keeping the patient sedated throughout the procedure. The postoperative lid height is very predictable with MMCR. Since the amount of resection is predetermined by the preoperative evaluation, there is no need for the patient's cooperation during the procedure and the patient can be sedated to ensure comfort.

A disadvantage of MMCR is that it does not address skin or crease abnormalities. It must be kept in mind that MMCR combined with an upper lid blepharoplasty leads to a lower postoperative height than expected. Dehiscence of the levator aponeurosis can result from increased swelling when both approaches are combined. Scarring between the anterior lamella of the eyelid and the levator complex is another plausible explanation for the reduction in predictable outcomes. Therefore, an anterior approach to ptosis repair with excision of excess skin and/or crease formation (see Chapter 6) is preferred in these cases.

TECHNIQUE

A frontal nerve block is given to avoid excessive intraoperative upper lid swelling: the needle is inserted, to a depth of approximately 4 mm, and 2 mL of 2% lidocaine with epinephrine (1:100,000) is injected 1 to 2 mm temporal to the supraorbital notch along the orbital roof. The central upper lid margin is infiltrated as well with 0.5 mL of the same anesthetic mixture. A 25-gauge retrobulbar-type needle is preferred for the block.

Complications from the frontal nerve block are retrobulbar hemorrhage and penetration of the globe. These risks are reduced if the surgeon uses a retrobulbar-type needle instead of a sharp needle and "hugs" the roof of the orbit when advancing the needle. Transient diplopia and mild to moderate blurring of vision can be seen in the immediate postoperative period secondary to the infiltration of the local anesthetic.

A 4-0 silk suture is placed through skin, orbicularis muscle, and partial thickness of the tarsus in the central upper lid margin for traction, while a Desmarres retractor is used to double-evert the lid and expose the tarsal and palpebral conjunctiva. As the eyelid is everted, the retractor typically sits on the superior border of the upper tarsus, blanching it and creating a readily identifiable line 8–10 mm from the lid margin, extending across the horizontal length of the lid on the conjunctival surface.

Calipers are used to measure and mark the predetermined amount of tissue to be resected above the superior border of the tarsus. With one arm of the caliper placed on the central superior tarsal border, the measurement is made in the superior palpebral conjunctiva. A double-armed 6-0 black silk suture is used to mark this point (Fig. 7.2).

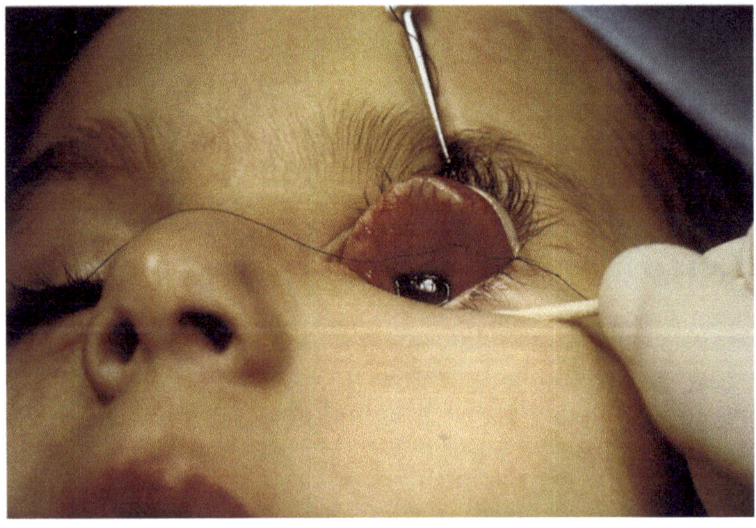

FIGURE 7.2. A double-armed 6-0 black silk suture is used to mark the superior palpebral conjunctiva.

   Muller's Muscle–Conjunctival Resection

Each end of the suture is then passed approximately 6 to 8 mm nasal and lateral to the central marking suture. A total of three suture bites are passed through the conjunctiva. Since this is only a temporary marking suture, which will make the next steps easier to perform, the type of suture is not important as long as it is readily visible.

Muller's muscle is loosely attached to the levator aponeurosis. These adhesions should be removed prior to tissue excision. The conjunctiva and Muller's muscle between the tarsal border and the marking suture are held with forceps and gently moved from side to side. This maneuver is repeated in different locations along the extent of the palpebral conjunctival surface. The release of Muller's muscle is partly responsible for the success of the following steps.

With the lid still everted, one of the blades of the toothed Muller's muscle–conjunctival resection clamp is placed just above the superior tarsal border (Fig. 7.3). The other blade is placed exactly over the marking suture. Before tightening, the surgeon should verify that conjunctiva under both blades is adequately engaged in the clamp. The enclosed tissues should contain only Muller's muscle and conjunctiva.

The key to success at this point is simultaneously closing the clamp and slowly removing the Desmarres retractor to prevent inclusion of

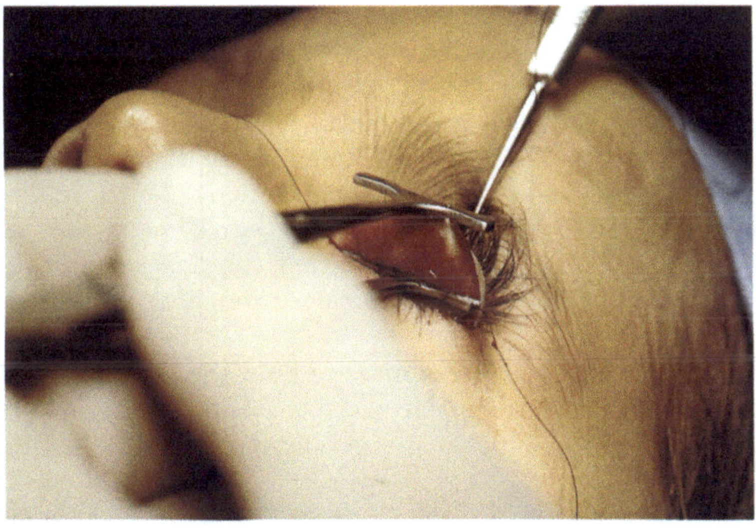

FIGURE 7.3. The blades of the resection clamp are placed just above the superior tarsal border, and exactly over the marking suture.

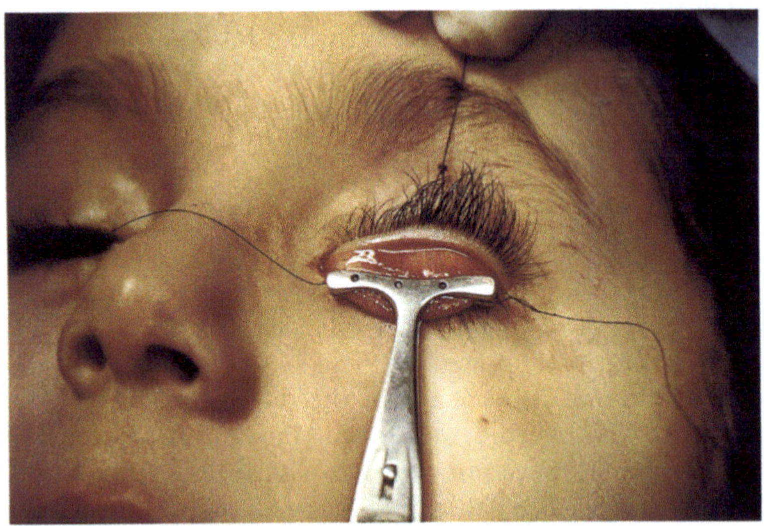

FIGURE 7.4. After removal of the Desmarres retractor, the clamp is closed without incorporating the overlying levator aponeurosis and skin.

the overlying levator aponeurosis and skin in the clamp (Fig. 7.4). The skin is gently pulled away from the clamped tissue with toothed forceps to confirm that the aponeurosis is not engaged. Remember that levator aponeurosis is tightly adherent to orbicularis and sends fibers through it into the skin to form the eyelid crease. Therefore if the anterior lamella of the eyelid (skin, orbicularis muscle, and levator aponeurosis) cannot be easily pulled away from the clamp, the clamp should be released, repositioned, and tightened again. Other situations that merit repositioning of the clamp are a poor grasp of conjunctiva and Muller's muscle on either the nasal or lateral sides, which may lead to potential undercorrection and a slanted eyelid contour.

The main purpose of the clamp is to hold the advanced tissues in place so that the surgeon can secure them before excision. A running double-armed 5-0 plain gut suture is placed in a horizontal mattress

Muller's Muscle–Conjunctival Resection

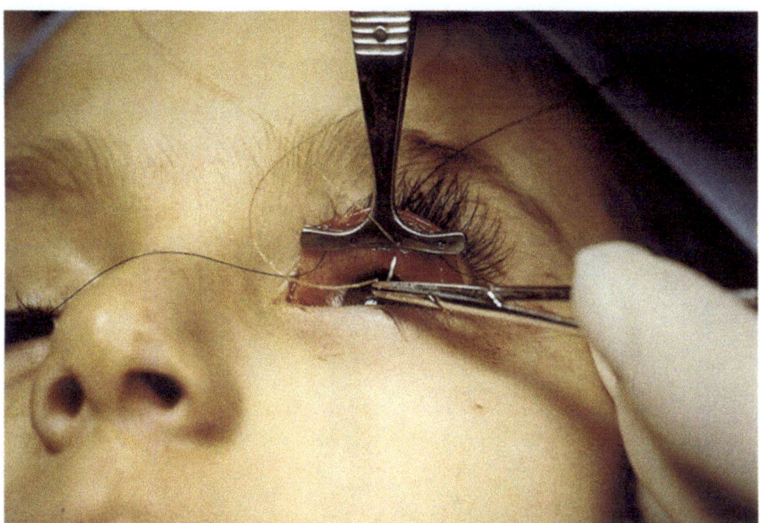

FIGURE 7.5. A double-armed 5-0 plain gut suture is run in a horizontal mattress fashion 1.5 mm beneath the clamp.

fashion 1.5 mm beneath the clamp (Fig. 7.5). It is essential to view the needle on both sides of the clamp, at entry and exit. This ensures its correct position and prevents accidentally cutting the suture in the next step. Plain gut is the suture of choice for this type of advancement, since it provides strength for the amount of time needed. More importantly, this suture is well tolerated by patients. Plain gut also produces a low-grade inflammation thought to be important for the scar formation needed to stabilize the advanced tissues. Vicryl, on the other hand, creates less inflammation, lasts too long, and is more uncomfortable to the patient. Nonabsorbable sutures can be harmful to the cornea and are contraindicated.

A #15 Bard–Parker blade is used to sever the tissue held by the clamp. The blade is placed between the horizontal mattress suture and the clamp. The surgeon angles the blade toward the clamp and begins the excision. As the blade is advanced, it maintains at all times

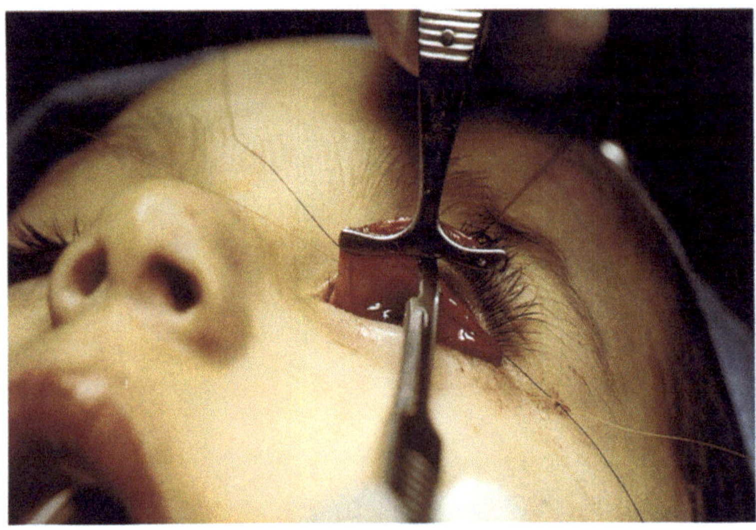

FIGURE 7.6. Clamp and excess tissue are removed as the blade is carefully advanced. The blade maintains a "metal-on-metal" position, to avoid cutting the preplaced gut suture.

a "metal-on-metal" position to avoid cutting the gut suture (Fig. 7.6). The silk marking suture is removed from the conjunctiva once the tissues have been resected. The surgeon may close the nasal conjunctiva with the gut suture in a running fashion, but this is usually not necessary.

Bleeding after the excision of the tissues can be significant and occasionally makes the closure of the conjunctiva difficult. Nevertheless hemostasis can be easily achieved with ice packs and gentle pressure.

The conjunctiva will rapidly close by itself. In the authors' experience, complete closure of the conjunctiva is not necessary. Instead, the last steps of the procedure may be modified to make the closure easier and more efficient for the surgeon, and better tolerated by the patient, since there is less suturing required and no knot. After the gut suture has been run under the clamp, both ends of the suture are brought full thickness through the eyelid, exiting on the skin surface. Tincture of benzoin and a small piece of surgical tape are used to hold the suture in place for 5 to 7 days.

Antibiotic ointment is applied to the eye for prophylaxis and lubrication at the end of the procedure and then 3 to 4 times daily for approximately a week. Mild postoperative bleeding is common and is

Muller's Muscle–Conjunctival Resection

easily controlled with gentle pressure and continuous ice packs in the early postoperative period. The patient should expect blood-tinged tears for approximately 48 hours and is instructed to use ice packs 15 minutes every hour for the first 48 to 72 waking hours, since edema of the eyelid usually resolves during this period. One week after the surgery the surgical tapes are removed, and the suture can be removed or the ends trimmed if necessary.

COMPLICATIONS

Most of the potential complications that can arise from MMCR are preventable if care is taken to get a detailed history and a meticulous preoperative evaluation.

Patients with known stable *cardiovascular disease* should be evaluated with 2.5% phenylephrine and punctual blockage for 3 to 5 min, rather than with 10% phenylephrine. Most surgeons consider alternative procedures of ptosis repair in *high-risk patients with known cerebral aneurysms, cerebrovascular disease, or severe coronary artery disease.*

Potential complications of the frontal nerve block are orbital hemorrhage and ocular penetration. "Hugging" the orbital roof with the needle and avoiding direct contact with the supraorbital neurovascular bundle prevent the surgeon from inadvertently penetrating the globe or causing orbital hemorrhage, respectively. Transient diplopia and blurred vision are not uncommon if the local anesthetic spreads to the intraconal space. However, orbital hemorrhage should always be high on the differential diagnosis and must be ruled out in the presence of any degree of visual decline after an orbital or periocular procedure.

Although uncommon, undercorrection is the most frequent complication of MMCR. This situation can result from improper placement of the marking suture or resection clamp, or slipping of the tissues from the clamp if it was not closed correctly. Undercorrection of approximately 1 mm can be expected when an MMCR is combined with an upper eyelid blepharoplasty, possibly owing to increased inflammation and swelling. An anterior approach is recommended when both excision of skin and ptosis repair are required.

Overcorrection with lagophthalmos is extremely rare. When punctate epithelial keratopathy develops, it is likely to be caused by the tarsal suture, not overcorrection. The cornea is treated with generous lubrication and usually resolves within a week after the suture dissolves. In the authors' experience, the self-sealing technique offers more comfort to the patient and decreases the chances of keratopathy. Also, many surgeons believe that if a knot is tied on the conjunctival surface, the incidence of keratopathy increases.

REFERENCES

1. Brown MS, Putterman AM. The effect of upper blepharoplasty on eyelid position when performed concomitantly with Muller muscle–conjunctival resection. *Ophthalmic Plast Reconstr Surg* 2000;16(2):94–100.

2. Dutton JJ. *Atlas of Ophthalmic Surgery.* Vol II. *Oculoplastic, Lacrimal and Orbital Surgery.* St. Louis: Mosby-Year Book; 1992.

3. Glatt HJ, Fett DR, Putterman AM. Comparison of the 2.5% and 10% phenylephrine in the elevation of upper eyelids with ptosis. *Ophthalmic Surg* 1990;21(3):173–176.

4. Glatt HJ, Putterman AM, Fett DR. Muller's muscle–conjunctival resection procedure in the treatment of ptosis in Horner's syndrome. *Ophthalmic Surg* 1990;21(2):93–96.

5. Karesh JW, Putterman AM, Fett DR. Conjunctiva–Muller's muscle excision to correct anophthalmic ptosis. *Ophthalmology* 1986;93(8):1068–1071.

6. Putterman AM, Fett DR. Muller's muscle in the treatment of upper eyelid ptosis: a ten-year study. *Ophthalmic Surg* 1986;17(6):354–360.

7. Putterman AM, Urist MJ. Muller muscle–conjunctiva resection. *Arch Ophthalmol* 1975;93:619–623.

8. Nesi FA, Gladstone GJ, Brazzo BG et al, eds. *Ophthalmic and Facial Plastic Surgery: A Compendium of Reconstructive and Aesthetic Techniques.* Thorofare, NJ: Slack Incorporated, 2000.

9. Weinstein GS, Buerger GF. Modifications of the Muller's muscle–conjunctival resection operation for blepharoptosis. *Am J Ophthalmol* 1982;93:647–651.

8

Small-Incision External Levator Repair

- Mark J. Lucarelli
- Briggs E. Cook, Jr.
- Bradley N. Lemke

In ophthalmology and other surgical subspecialties there is a progressive movement toward minimally invasive surgery.[1] The goals of small-incision surgery include decreased morbidity, tissue preservation, decreased operative time, rapid healing, and reduced scarring. Minimizing dissection in blepharoptosis surgery offers several advantages. Reduced edema and bleeding and less local anesthetic allow more accurate assessment of eyelid position and function intraoperatively. This chapter discusses a technique for small-incision external levator repair of aponeurogenic blepharoptosis.[2]

EVALUATION

The preoperative evaluation should begin with a careful history. Patients with visually significant blepharoptosis frequently present with complaints of "drooping" eyelids, difficulty with superotemporal visual field, trouble reading signs while driving, and fatigue while reading. Patients are also frequently aware of brow ache or frontalis flexion resulting from brow recruitment. A history of diplopia might suggest a myogenic or neurological process such as chronic progressive external ophthalmoplegia or myasthenia gravis. A careful history about dry eye symptoms and the use of artificial tears should also be obtained. Such information frequently modifies the surgical plan. In the general medical history, any anticoagulant medications or drugs that inhibit platelet function should be carefully noted.

A complete ophthalmic examination is appropriate prior to ptosis surgery. Particular attention should be paid to the condition of the ocular surface, the quality of the tear film, and the height of the tear meniscus. These signs will help identify patients with undiagnosed dry eye who are at risk for exposure keratopathy or worsening of their dry eye condition postoperatively. If the history or examination suggests a problem with dry eye, a Schirmer's test is appropriate to quantify the tear production. Basic eyelid measurements such as margin reflex distances, levator excursion, and lagophthalmos are routine. The authors have generally reserved this small-incision external levator repair for patients with levator excursion measuring 8 mm or more. A poor Bell's phenomenon should be noted, as this indicates poor postoperative tolerance of any lagophthalmus. Similarly, poor lower lid position should be noted and corrected at the time of the ptosis surgery or beforehand.

Additionally, upper lid horizontal laxity and lateral canthal dehiscence should be noted. Identifying and addressing these eyelid changes help to improve the results of ptosis surgery and reduce postoperative complications. Failure to address excessive upper eyelid laxity or lateral canthal dehiscence (such as seen in floppy eyelid syndrome) makes it difficult to achieve proper upper eyelid contour. The authors frequently employ a small-incision, canthus-sparing lateral canthopexy[3] (described shortly) intraoperatively in such cases.

An accurate assessment of dermatochalasis in the upper eyelids is crucial prior to recommending small-incision levator repair. The authors generally reserve this technique for patients with minimal to mild dermatochalasis (0–1 on a scale of 4). If concurrent upper blepharoplasty is indicated, the small-incision levator repair may be performed through the orbital septum. If significant lash ptosis is present, standard ptosis repair that allows correction of lash ptosis across the entire eyelid is recommended.

Assessment of the eyebrow position with the frontalis musculature relaxed is also crucial. Failure to evaluate the patient's eyelids while the brow is relaxed can result in underestimation of the degree of dermatochalasis or brow ptosis. Such an error in preoperative evaluation will compromise the final result, indicating that browlift or blepharoplasty should have been performed as an adjunctive procedure. The authors' only disappointing results with this technique postoperatively have resulted from underappreciation of dermatochalasis or brow ptosis preoperatively.

TECHNIQUE

Local infiltrative anesthesia is utilized with monitored sedation with propofol (Diprivan, Zeneca Pharmaceuticals, Wilmington, DE). A surgical marking pen is used to delineate the upper eyelid crease at the appropriate horizontal position to achieve the best eyelid margin contour. The original description of this technique[2] recommended an 8 mm incision. Two of the authors (BNL and BEC) continue to favor this incision length. The horizontal position of the incision site is carefully determined by elevating the eyelid with a cotton-tipped applicator or forceps at various positions along the lid crease and observing the eyelid contour.

In a minor modification of this small-incision technique, some surgeons use a 12 mm incision, generally extending from the medial corneal limbus to the lateral corneal limbus. This slight lengthening of the incision increases exposure, facilitates isolation of the levator aponeurosis and placement of multiple tarsal sutures, and generally preserves the small-incision advantages of the technique. Approximately 0.6 mL of 2% lidocaine with 1:200,000 units of epinephrine is injected into the eyelid.

The skin incision is made with straight iris scissors or other instrument. Dissection through the orbicularis is performed with a microdissection needle (Colorado Biomedical, Evergreen, CO), driven by a monopolar electrosurgical unit. The superior half of the tarsus is exposed for a length of 10 to 12 mm.

With the assistant providing traction in an inferior and anterior direction, the surgeon grasps the preseptal orbicularis and retracts superiorly. The orbital septum is incised above its point of fusion with the levator complex. The preaponeurotic fat pad is identified and retracted superiorly (Fig. 8.1). Blunt dissection is carried superiorly along the anterior surface of the levator complex to a point several millimeters above the level of the musculoaponeurotic junction. The terminal aspect of the levator aponeurosis is generally dehiscent, and additional dissection between the aponeurosis and Muller's muscle is generally not required.

Eyelid contour is again carefully assessed by elevating the tarsus at various horizontal positions immediately prior to placement of the tarsal suture(s). After the ideal position for suturing has been determined, a spatulated needle on a 5-0 nylon suture (Ethicon #7731, Somerville, NJ) is directed partial thickness through the tarsus in a horizontal fashion. The needle is next directed superiorly underneath the levator complex and retrieved on the anterior surface of the lev-

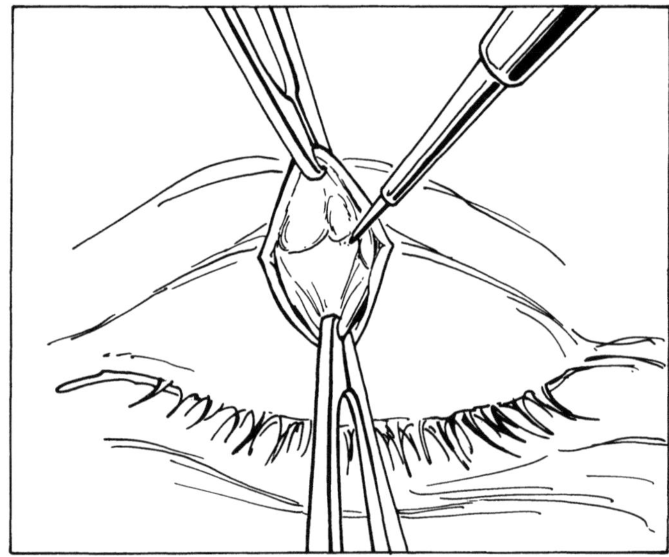

FIGURE 8.1. The preaponeurotic fat pad is identified and the anterior surface of the levator complex is exposed to a point several millimeters above the musculoaponeurotic junction. (Reproduced with permission from Lucarelli MJ, Lemke BN. Small incision external levator repair: technique and early results. *Am J Ophthalmol* 1999;127:637–644.)

Small-Incision External Levator Repair

ator complex slightly above the musculoaponeurotic junction or just below Whitnall's transverse ligament. A surgeon's knot is placed, and the suture loop is partially tightened to provide an appropriate degree of lift (Fig. 8.2).

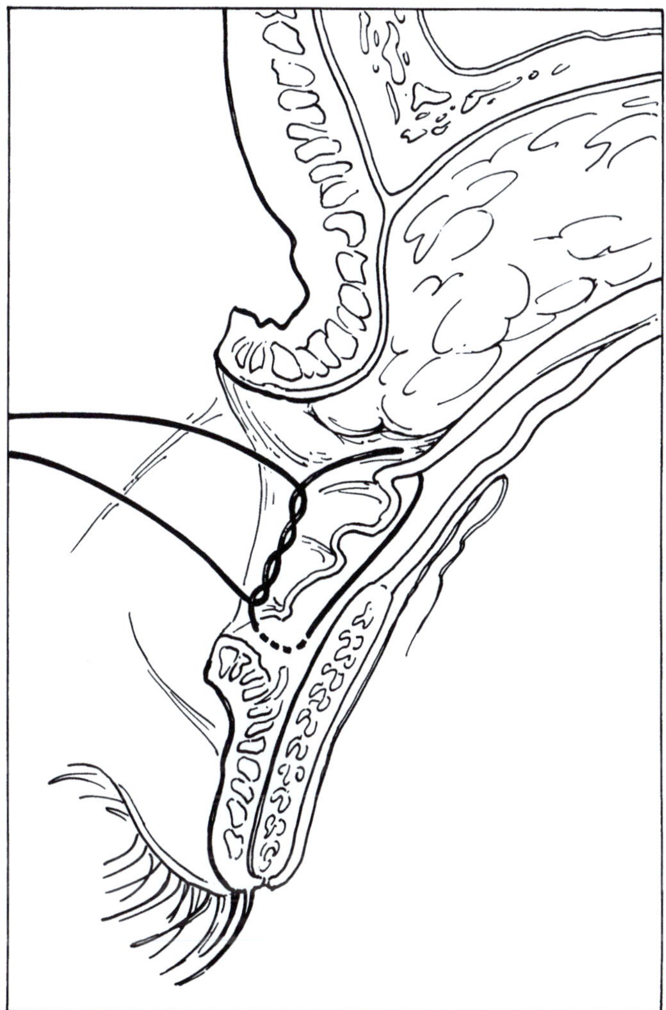

FIGURE 8.2. The suture is adjusted to provide the desired eyelid height. (Reproduced with permission from Lucarelli MJ, Lemke BN. Small incision external levator repair: technique and early results. *Am J Ophthalmol* 1999;127:637–644.)

Ten minutes prior to intraoperative assessment of eyelid position, the intravenous propofol is discontinued to allow accurate intraoperative assessment. Eyelid height and contour are inspected in primary gaze, upgaze, and downgaze. The suture is tightened or loosened as necessary. The suture loop is next tied at the desired length over a needle holder. Medial and lateral supplemental sutures may be placed on either side of the cardinal suture in an identical fashion at the surgeon's discretion.

Alternatively, the tarsal sutures may be placed in a horizontal mattress fashion, passing initially through the levator aponeurosis from anterior to posterior, then horizontally through the tarsus before again penetrating the levator aponeurosis. With this method, redundant levator aponeurosis may be excised as desired. A 6-0 Prolene suture is also suitable for the levator–tarsal suture.

Eyelid crease re-formation is not necessary or desired with this technique. The orbicularis may be closed with one or two 7-0 Vicryl interrupted subcuticular sutures. The skin is closed in a running fashion by using 6-0 fast-absorbing gut suture (Fig. 8.3).

The principles of this technique may also be utilized and some of the benefits achieved in the setting of ptosis repair combined with upper blepharoplasty. In such cases, the blepharoplasty is performed in a standard fashion. Subsequently, the external levator repair is performed. However, only the central 10 to 12 mm of the orbital septum and the tarsus are dissected. The lateral and medial aspects of the levator are left undisturbed. With less dissection of the levator, less local anesthetic is needed, and less bleeding and intraoperative edema occur. These factors help to make determination of the intraoperative endpoint more accurate even in the setting of an open blepharoplasty incision. Less mobilization of the levator aponeurosis seems to reduce problems with postoperative eyelid contour.

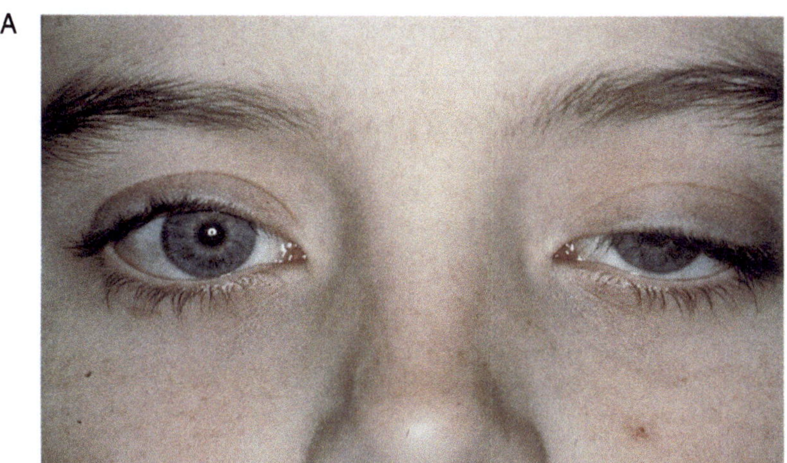

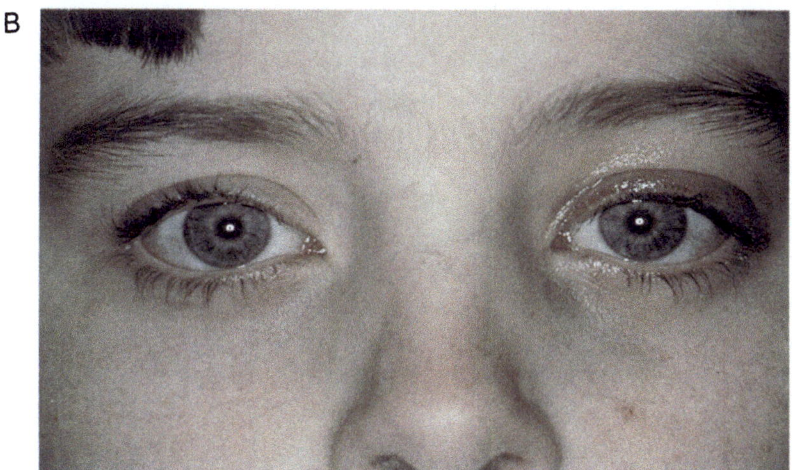

FIGURE 8.3. (A) Congenital ptosis with 10 mm levator excursion. (B) Four-day postoperative result following small incision technique, with minimal edema.

Adjunctive Lateral Canthopexy with Small-Incision External Levator Repair

When significant lateral canthal dehiscence or upper eyelid laxity is present, external levator repair may be improved by performing adjunctive lateral canthopexy.[4] With this variation the small-incision external levator repair is performed as described earlier to the point of isolating the levator aponeurosis. Attention is then directed to the lateral palpebral raphe. A 6 to 8 mm incision is made lateral to the lateral canthus. A lateral canthotomy is not created. Dissection is then continued with the microdissection needle through the orbital portion of the orbicularis muscle to reach the lateral orbital rim.

While the incision is held apart with fingertips or four-pronged rakes, a posteriorly based, 7×3 mm^2 periosteal flap is created on the anterior aspect of the lateral orbital rim. The periosteal flap is raised with a Freer elevator to a point 3 mm inside the lateral orbital rim at the level of Whitnall's lateral orbital tubercle. The generous vertical dimension of the flap helps to minimize shredding of the flap during dissection and suturing.

Next a 5-0 Prolene suture on a PS-5 needle (Ethicon) is used to grasp the common crus of the lateral canthal tendon. Adequate tissue purchase is confirmed with traction on the suture. Tightly linked movement of the lateral canthal tendon should be observed. The suture is then passed full thickness through the periosteal flap inside the lateral orbital rim. Tension is adjusted on the suture, and it is tied in a permanent fashion. Upon reestablishment of appropriate horizontal tension along the upper eyelid, the small-incision external levator repair is completed as described earlier.

COMPLICATIONS

The small incision in this technique has several advantages as already described. The small incision length does not prevent adequate surgical exposure, although reduced exposure can make identifying the levator complex more challenging. As with other periocular procedures, a solid knowledge of anatomy is paramount. The current technique evolved by gradually reducing the incision length. This is probably a reasonable approach for most surgeons who perform ptosis surgery rather than moving directly from a full upper eyelid incision to an 8 mm incision. In the event that the levator complex proves difficult to isolate through an 8 mm incision, the upper eyelid crease incision can easily be extended to a intermediate or standard length.

In any variation of external levator repair, judging the endpoint of the upper eyelid height can be challenging.[5] It can be especially problematic when excessive edema or hemorrhage occurs intraoperatively. Similar difficulty occurs when the local anesthetic has the unintended effect of reducing levator excursion. In such rare cases, the levator–tarsus sutures are secured with a surgeon's knot, trimmed at approximately 15 to 20 mm, and left exposed outside the wound to allow adjustment in the early postoperative period. When the authors have utilized this technique, adjustment is performed at approximately 3 to 4 days postoperatively in the office. Such an adjustment can usually be done with topical anesthetic only.

Like other forms of external levator repair, postoperative undercorrection or overcorrection is possible with this technique. In the authors' initial experience with small-incision external levator repair, two of 28 (7%) eyelids were undercorrected by slightly more than 1 mm.[2] No eyelid was overcorrected. Residual ptosis may be corrected in the office under local anesthetic after postoperative edema has been minimized and levator function has returned to its preoperative state (almost always by 7–10 days).

Eyelid contour abnormalities can generally be avoided by paying careful attention to the horizontal placement of the levator–tarsal suture(s). Identifying and correcting horizontal laxity of the upper eyelid also reduce the likelihood of postoperative contour problems. In the original description, one of 28 (4%) eyelids demonstrated moderately peaked contour.

Proper preoperative selection of patients is especially important in this technique. Patients with only minimal to mild dermatochalasis are considered good candidates. Those with moderate to severe dermatochalasis generally benefit from skin–muscle blepharoplasty in conjunction with external levator repair. Even in patients undergoing an upper blepharoplasty, the small incision of the orbital septum may be employed to minimize dissection at the level of the levator aponeurosis and the tarsus.

Underestimation of brow ptosis can be problematic. In some patients with severe blepharoptosis, continuous marked frontalis flexion may hide a relatively severe brow ptosis. Such frontalis flexion also can conceal significant dermatochalasis. When the dermatochalasis or brow ptosis is underestimated, the result will be suboptimal.

Acknowledgment
This work was supported by an unrestricted grant from Research to Prevent Blindness, Inc., New York, New York.

REFERENCES

1. Dortzbach RK, Woog JJ. Small-incision techniques in ophthalmic plastic surgery. *Ophthalmic Surg* 1990;21:615–622.

2. Lucarelli MJ, Lemke BN. Small incision external levator repair: technique and early results. *Am J Ophthalmol* 1999;127:637–644.

3. Lemke BN, Cook BE, Lucarelli MJ. Canthus-sparing ectropion repair. *Ophthalmic Plast Reconstr Surg* 2001;17(3):161–168.

4. Shore JW, Neuhaus RW, Blaydon S. Correcting upper eyelid horizontal laxity during ptosis repair. Presented at the 1998 American Society of Ophthalmic Plastic and Reconstructive Surgery (ASOPRS) Fall Symposium, New Orleans.

5. Dortzbach RK, Gausas RA, Sherman DD. Blepharoptosis. In: Dortzbach RK, ed. *Ophthalmic Plastic Surgery: Prevention and Management of Complications.* New York: Raven; 1994:70–71.

PART III

LOWER EYELID MALPOSITION

9

Subperiosteal Midface Lift

• Julian D. Perry
• Norman Shorr

Typically, postblepharoplasty lower eyelid retraction involves a combination of anterior, middle, and posterior vertical lamellar inadequacy. The degree of inadequacy of each individual layer of the eyelid must be evaluated, and its relationship to the underlying bony rim projection and globe prominence must be defined. Patients are often not satisfied with the lower eyelid aesthetics and have symptoms of corneal exposure. They demonstrate inferior scleral show, with rounding and dystopia of the lateral canthal angle.

EVALUATION

The digital elevation test (shown in Chapter 12: Fig. 12.1) aids in defining the degree of middle lamellar cicatrix. The examiner places a forefinger on the lower eyelid and attempts to push the lower lid superiorly. Normally, the lower lid can be raised above the superior limbus. Significant cicatrix exists when the lid cannot be raised to this level. Frequently following blepharoplasty or other surgery, the eyelid cannot be raised to the level of the midpupil.

The surgeon must isolate the level of cicatrix. To evaluate the degree of anterior lamellar insufficiency, the examiner asks the patient to open his or her mouth. This maneuver places the anterior lamella on stretch. Patients with significant anterior lamellar insufficiency demonstrate inferior movement of the lid margin upon opening the mouth. Posterior (conjunctival) cicatrix is uncommon and can be directly observed by pulling the eyelid inferiorly, away from the globe. A shallow fornix and symblepharon formation are clues to posterior etiology.

If the symptomatic patient has had lower eyelid surgery or trauma, and if skin and conjunctiva appear to be adequate, the surgeon can be comfortable with a diagnosis of middle lamellar cicatrix. However, there may be scarring within more than one layer that is not detected during the initial examination. These tests should be repeated intraoperatively as well. When the primary cicatrix is released, a second layer of scar may become apparent and should be treated appropriately.

Slit lamp evaluation after instillation of sodium fluoroscein into the conjunctival cul-de-sac often reveals signs of exposure keratopathy, including punctate epithelial erosions, conjunctival injection, and a decreased tear meniscus.

Counseling patients and deciding when to repair the retraction are critical steps in management. Although patients typically desire immediate resolution, the surgeon must understand the healing process and treat accordingly. Eyelid retraction typically reaches its peak between postoperative weeks 3 and 8. The tissues may gradually soften and relax over the next several months. During this period, the patient requires frequent encouragement and office visits.

Often, the surgeon may institute maneuvers designed to manipulate the healing process. If a discrete area of cicatrix can be palpated on digital elevation testing, low dose triamcinolone (10 mg/mL, approximately 0.1–0.5 mL) may be injected into the region. The patient should also be instructed to massage the eyelids, which may relax the tether. The patient places a forefinger just beneath the lid margin in the area of maximal tether and pushes the eyelid superiorly for 10 seconds, relaxes for several seconds, then pushes superiorly again. The patient may perform 10 repetitions four times daily. Lid massage gives one a constructive way to help the condition during the waiting period.

If the tether, subsequent aesthetic deformity, or symptoms of exposure have not resolved after 4 to 6 months of conservative management, the surgeon and patient must decide whether to proceed with surgical aesthetic reconstructive options. The complexity of the repair and realistic surgical goals should be discussed. Many surgeons offer a "minor" procedure, such as lateral canthoplasty, to elevate the lower lid. However, procedures such as this may not address the underlying anatomic and structural deformities. Sub–orbicularis oculi fat (SOOF) lifting with lateral canthoplasty and posterior lamellar grafting frequently achieves successful cosmetic and functional results while avoiding a skin graft. Typically, the greater the middle lamellar tether and anterior lamellar inadequacy, the more challenging the repair.

TECHNIQUE

Surgical repair is aimed at reconstructing all three individual layers of the eyelid, and augmenting the orbital rim and subrim projection when appropriate. The posterior lamella is reconstructed with placement of a graft between the inferior tarsal border and the recessed lower lid retractors and conjunctiva. The middle lamellar cicatrix is lysed and then splinted by a posterior lamellar graft of hard palate or acellular human dermal matrix tissue. Elevating the underlying SOOF augments the anterior lamella. The lower eyelid is temporarily supported by suturing the lower lid margin to the upper lid margin and finally to the eyebrow.

The zygomaticus and levator labii superioris alaeque nasi muscles are quite vascular. Therefore, adequate local infiltration of an epinephrine-containing solution is critical for hemostasis. Under local standby anesthesia, all surgical areas are infiltrated with a solution containing 2% lidocaine with epinephrine (1:100,000) and hyaluronidase. The entire lower eyelid and cheek must be infiltrated to achieve adequate hemostasis. A supraorbital nerve block is also recommended.

Prior to making an incision, superior traction testing is performed with 0.5 mm forceps to determine the degree of middle lamellar cicatrix. This test is repeated frequently throughout the procedure to

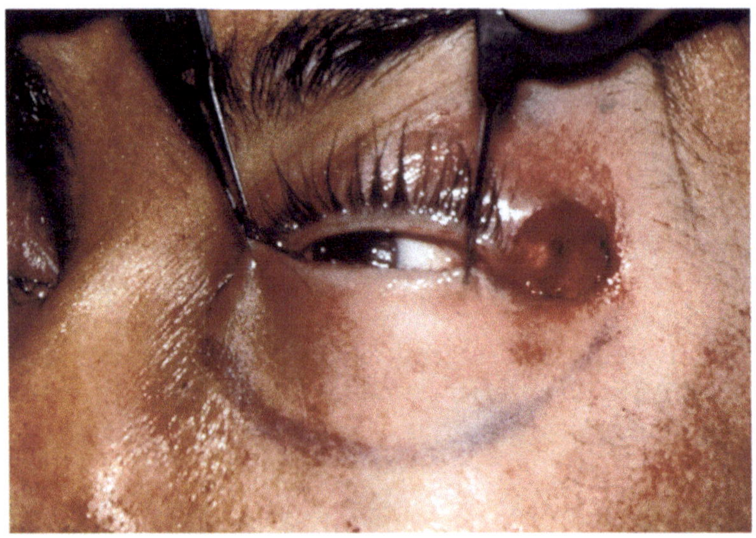

FIGURE 9.1. Middle lamellar cicatrix prevents surgeon from elevating the lower lid past the mid-pupil.

determine the degree to which the middle lamellar cicatrix has been lysed (Figs. 9.1 and 9.2).

After lateral canthotomy and cantholysis, the bony lateral rim is exposed. The authors typically mark the lateral rim with the monopo-

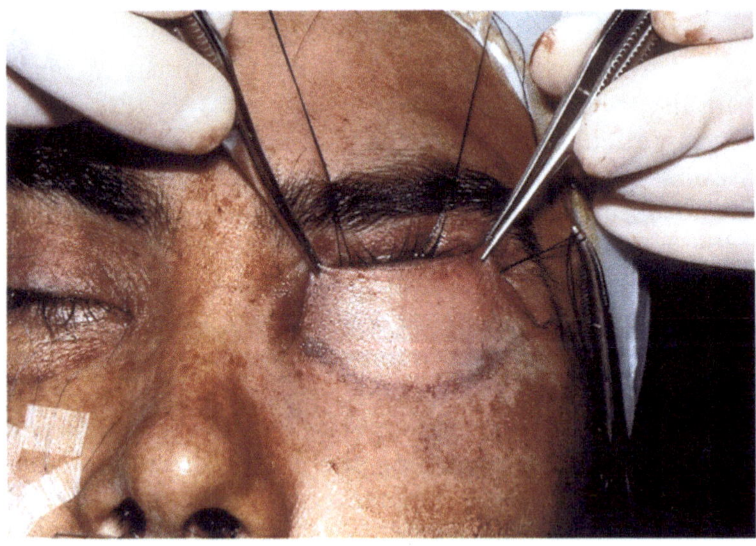

FIGURE 9.2. After surgical release of the middle lamellar cicatrix, the eyelid easily elevates with superior traction.

lar cautery at the level of the lateral canthal angle if no preexisting lateral canthal dystopia exists. This maneuver will assist in repositioning the lateral canthal angle at the appropriate height toward the end of the procedure. If the angle is dystopic and low, the authors mark the periosteum to approximate the correct position of the angle to facilitate later repositioning of the angle.

The conjunctiva and lower eyelid retractors are incised just beneath tarsus along the entire horizontal extent of the lower eyelid. It is important to carry this incision sufficiently medially through the caruncle to allow exposure in this area. The dissection along the posterior surface of the septum inferiorly to the arcus marginalis should lyse the middle lamellar tether with a combination of blunt and sharp dissection.

The assistant retracts the anterior lower lid with a Desmarres retractor while the surgeon grasps the conjunctiva with 0.5 mm Castroviejo forceps to place the middle lamella on stretch. The cicatricial tether is visualized as "bands" running in the anterior–posterior plane (Fig. 9.3). Blunt dissection with a cotton-tipped applicator allows a precise way to define this plane, although the larger bands must be lysed sharply. Care should be taken to avoid piercing the septum and exposing the orbital fat during this dissection to the bony rim. Pro-

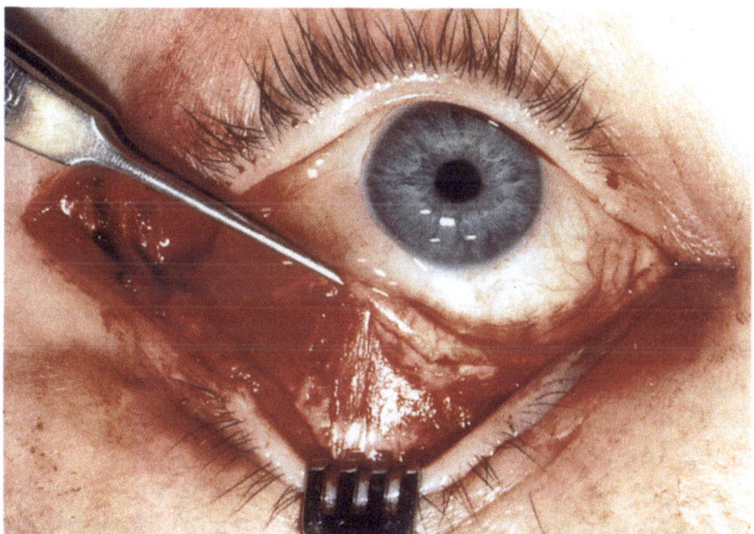

FIGURE 9.3. The cicatricial tether is visualized as bands running in the anterior–posterior plane. This tether must be lysed with a combination of sharp and blunt dissection.

lapsed orbital fat will make placement of the suspension sutures somewhat more difficult and increase the risk of postoperative scarring.

After lysis of the middle lamellar cicatrix, the arcus marginalis is incised by means of monopolar cautery approximately 2 mm inferior to the inferior orbital rim. This incision creates a superior cuff of periosteum that will later be used to suspend the SOOF. This cuff of periosteum tends to retract somewhat, so care must be taken to create enough tissue to allow for a good purchase with the cheek suspension sutures.

Several important points must be addressed when one is beginning the subperiosteal dissection. Medially, just anterior to the anterior lacrimal crest, the surgeon frequently encounters bleeding from the bone in the area of the sutura notha. Reinfiltration medially, in the area of the levator labii superioris alaeque nasi muscle, prior to subperiosteal dissection in this area, will aid in hemostasis.

The subperiosteal dissection centrally, in the area of the levator labii superioris alaeque nasi, should similarly begin with caution. Because the muscle runs directly over the infraorbital foramen, careful dissection here will avoid injury to these neurovascular structures. Care should be taken to avoid excessive cautery in this area, which may cause nerve damage and persistent postoperative pain. Laterally, the subperiosteal dissection proceeds to masseteric muscle fibers. Because branches of the facial nerve run directly over the masseter muscle and zygoma, special care must be taken to remain in the subperiosteal plane laterally.

Following complete dissection, an inferior periosteotomy is performed. While scissors, a finger, or a periosteal elevator may be used for this maneuver, careful monopolar cautery offers the advantages of hemostasis and a more accurate incision. Care must be taken to incise only the periosteum, especially laterally, to avoid facial nerve branch injury. Medially, the incision begins over the lateral aspect of the nose. Centrally, the incision should proceed just superior to the buccal sulcus. To more adequately mobilize the cheek after the periosteotomy has been performed, a curved periosteal elevator is then introduced under the flap and used to bluntly separate the periosteum across the incision.

The authors have found several maneuvers that assist in adequately suspending the SOOF to the superior cuff of periosteum (Fig. 9.4). Typically, five or six suspension sutures are placed across the inferior and lateral orbital rim. Nonabsorbable suture such as 3-0 Pro-

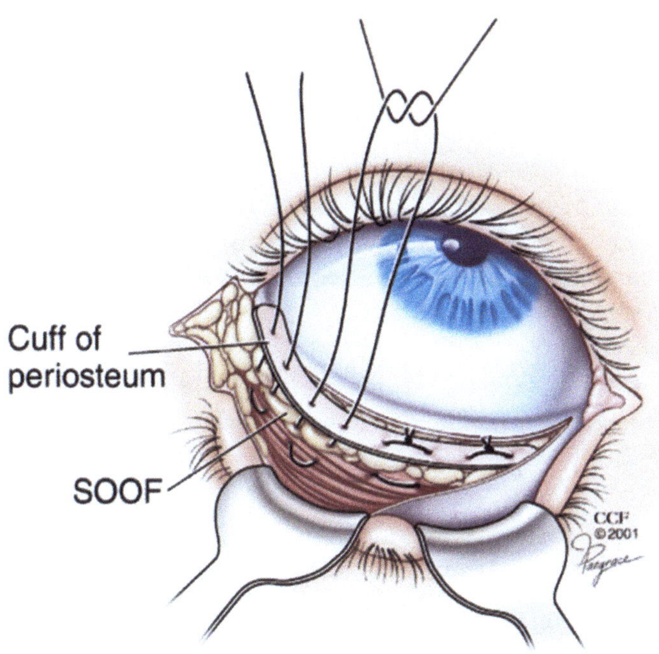

FIGURE 9.4. Multipoint fixation of the SOOF to the superior cuff of periosteum allows adequate anterior lamellar augmentation of the entire horizontal extent of the eyelid. (Created by Mark Sabo, Cleveland Clinic Foundation, with permission.)

lene and absorbable suture such as 3-0 PDS appear to give similar results.

The SOOF is grasped with forceps at various points on its superior margin and raised superiorly, to determine the desired vector of suspension. At each fixation point, the surgeon must grasp enough tissue to allow adequate suspension without causing dimpling of the overlying skin. If dimpling occurs, a deeper layer of SOOF is grasped with the forceps and the skin examined again. This maneuver is repeated until the appropriate degree and vector of lift are achieved without cutaneous irregularities. The surgeon then purchases this designated area of SOOF tissue with the needle, controlling the tissue with the forceps at all times while suspending it to the cuff of periosteum in mattress fashion. Before the suture is tied, the skin is again examined for dimpling with the suture pulled taut.

The authors use a half-circle needle to allow for easier purchase of the SOOF. This is especially important laterally, where the cheek must be suspended sufficiently superiorly along the lateral orbital periosteum. The authors sometimes bend the needle to a greater degree to allow easier suture placement in this area. Each suture is placed in mattress fashion, with the knot resting superior to the superior cuff of periosteum. If the suture knots appear to loosen after the first throw, the assistant may grasp the knot with a small-jawed needle driver to allow the second throw to achieve appropriate tension. Nonabsorbable sutures are cut short to decrease the likelihood of postoperative discomfort or palpation of the suture knots through the thin overlying tissues.

The appropriate horizontal length of the eyelid is then determined by draping the lower eyelid across the proposed site of the new lateral canthal angle. The gray line is excised in the area of horizontal shortening, and a "tongue" of tarsus (lateral tarsal strip) is created. The new position of lateral canthal angle is marked with a marking pen. A double-armed 5-0 Dexon suture on a half-circle needle, placed through the tarsal edge, can be used to stabilize the edge of tarsus during placement of a posterior lamellar graft. The suture ends are later placed through the periosteum of the inner aspect of the lateral orbital rim at the appropriate level, to complete the mattress stitch (Fig. 9.5). This suture is securely tied after the confirming that the lower eyelid reconstruction is complete.

When a hard palate graft is being used, several important points should be addressed before the lateral canthus is closed. A greater palatine nerve block is achieved by infiltrating 0.5 mL of 2% lidocaine with epinephrine (1:100,000) medial to the distal half of the last molar. When given correctly, the entire area of distribution of this nerve will blanch within several minutes of injection. The donor site is marked with a marking pencil on the hard palate laterally. The donor site should be parallel to and approximately 4 mm from the teeth. A graft from this area is smoother than a graft harvested toward the midline.

A typical graft may be 25 mm in length, tapering in width from 5 mm to 2 mm. The incision is made to a depth of approximately 2 mm along both sides of the graft with a #15 Bard–Parker blade. The

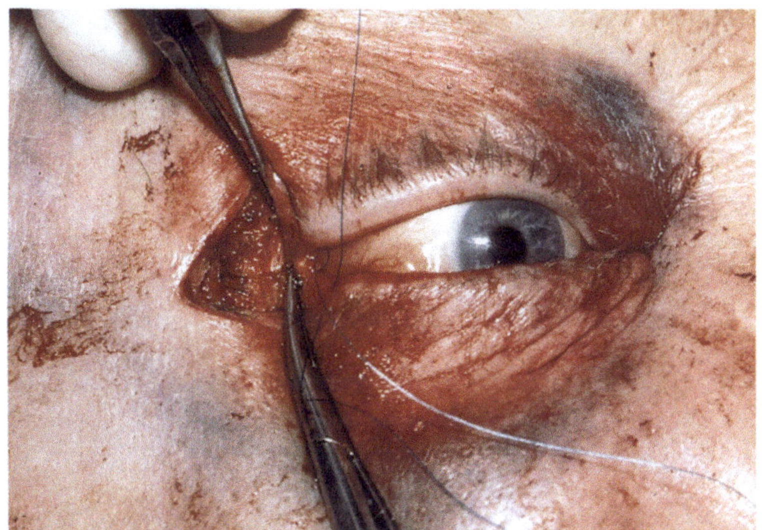

FIGURE 9.5. Preplacement of the lateral canthal resuspension suture reapproximates the tarsal strip to the inner aspect of the lateral orbital rim. This suture is tied only after placement of the posterior lamellar graft.

blade is used to undermine the graft just below the submucosal plane. Deep posterior dissection risks injury to the greater palatine artery, which may produce brisk bleeding. The graft is stored in sterile, moistened 4×4 gauze. Any areas of punctate bleeding may be lightly cauterized, and Coe-Pac periodontal paste or Surgi-Cel may be used to fill the defect. A prefit surgical impression plate is coated with dental adhesive and pressed against the hard palate, covering the donor site.

The hard palate graft is trimmed and thinned if necessary. The graft is placed so that its mucosal surface lies against the mucosal surface of the tarsal plate. Sutures should be placed to avoid contact with the cornea. Postoperative eye pain is most commonly due to corneal abrasion by a suture. A running buried 6-0 mild chromic suture is used to stabilize the posterior edges of the graft to tarsus. The graft is then rotated into the anatomical position, and a series of

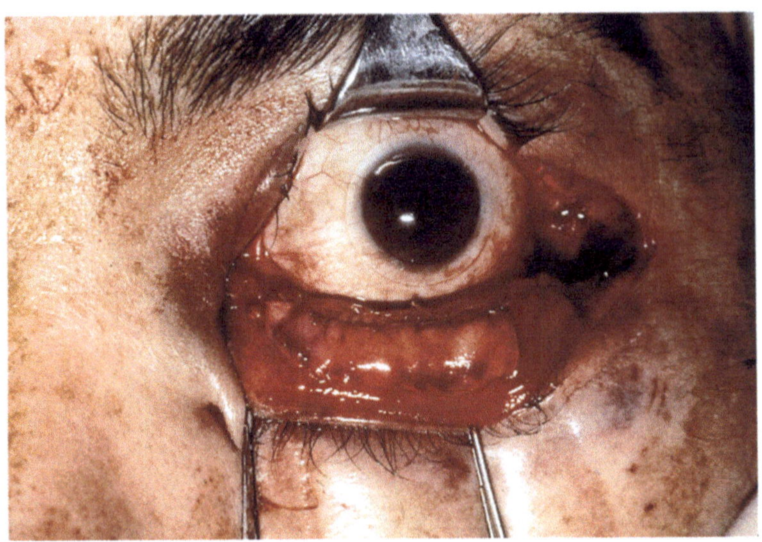

FIGURE 9.6. In situ placement of a posterior lamellar graft, secured in position with absorbable suture. Note the contact lens over the cornea. For this patient, acellular human dermal matrix tissue was used.

buried, interrupted 6-0 mild chromic sutures are passed from the conjunctival flap through the graft and tied (Fig. 9.6).

If suture material abrades the cornea, the patient may complain of severe postoperative discomfort. Treatment may require premature removal of the Frost suture for examination and excision of the offending suture, which may compromise the final surgical result. To avoid this complication, all sutures must be buried. The authors also place a bandage soft contact lens to protect the cornea postoperatively.

Acellular human dermal matrix tissue (AlloDerm, Life Cell Corp., The Woodlands, TX) may be a viable alternative to autogenous hard palate tissue as a posterior lamellar graft. Acellular human dermal matrix tissue is a commercially available product that avoids donor site morbidity. It is derived from human cadavers and is supplied in individually wrapped, freeze-dried packages. The material retains a basement membrane complex that may facilitate reepithelialization. This basement membrane surface should face the globe after placement. The material must be rehydrated according the manufacture's recommendations. It is easier to fashion the material before rehydration, although final trimming in situ is easily and frequently per-

   Subperiosteal Midface Lift

formed. The authors suture the material in the host bed just as in a
hard palate graft. The basement membrane surface is coarse and dull
and should face the cornea after placement. The reticular dermis side
of the graft should face the host bed.

After placement of the posterior lamellar graft, the lateral canthal angle is re-formed and resuspended. This step is critical to the
final aesthetic result, and several important points should be kept in
mind. The lateral canthal angle is re-formed by means of a mattress
suture of 6-0 mild chromic gut. Occasionally, a circular suture of 6-0
mild chromic gut through the gray line of both the upper and lower
lid is used in addition to the mattress suture to achieve a tight angle (lateral commissure). The angle is more easily approximated before tightening and securing the suture that was previously placed
from the tarsal strip to the lateral bony rim.

After the canthal angle has been re-formed, the horizontal mattress suture is drawn up and tied (Fig. 9.7). This critical suture determines the height of the lateral canthal angle. Most patients will
complain of noticeable deformity if this suture is not properly placed.

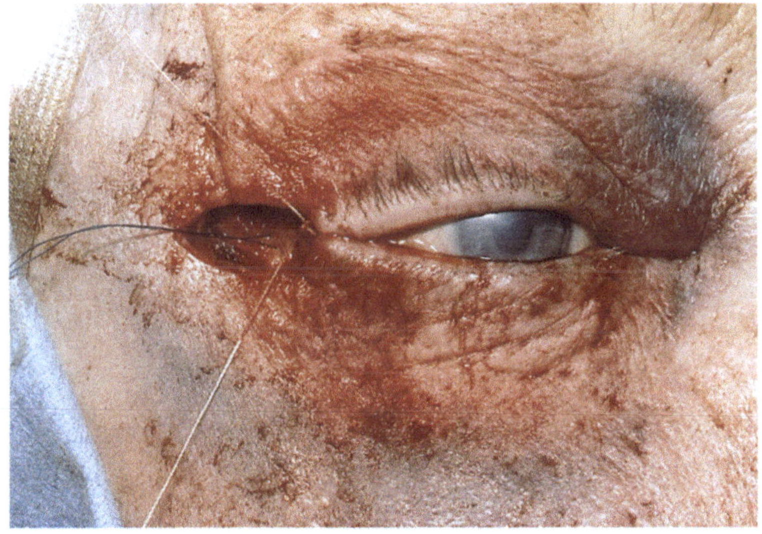

FIGURE 9.7. Final tying of the lateral canthal resuspension
suture and the lateral commissure suture. The patient should
sit upright prior to final tying to assure excellent position of
the angle.

After initial placement, the patient should be placed in the upright position to reevaluate the position of the angle. The suture should be adjusted until appropriate position of the angle is achieved. Several orbicularis suspension sutures of 5-0 Dexon are used to stabilize the orbicularis to the periosteum overlying the zygoma lateral to the lateral orbital rim. The cutaneous incision of the lateral canthotomy may be closed with a running 6-0 mild chromic suture.

A Frost suture is then placed to keep the lid on stretch during the early postoperative period. Three 6-0 Prolene horizontal mattress sutures are passed from the eyebrow, through the upper eyelid margin, along the gray line of the lower eyelid margin, then back through the eyebrow and tied on themselves. These three sutures are drawn to adequate tension to support the lower eyelid during the first week of healing. Typically, adequate tension is achieved when the lower lid margin rests at the level of the superior pupil. The eyelids are dressed with ophthalmic antibiotic–steroid ointment and casted with two eye patches, Mastisol, and paper tape. The cast may be removed 5 to 7 days postoperatively (Fig. 9.8).

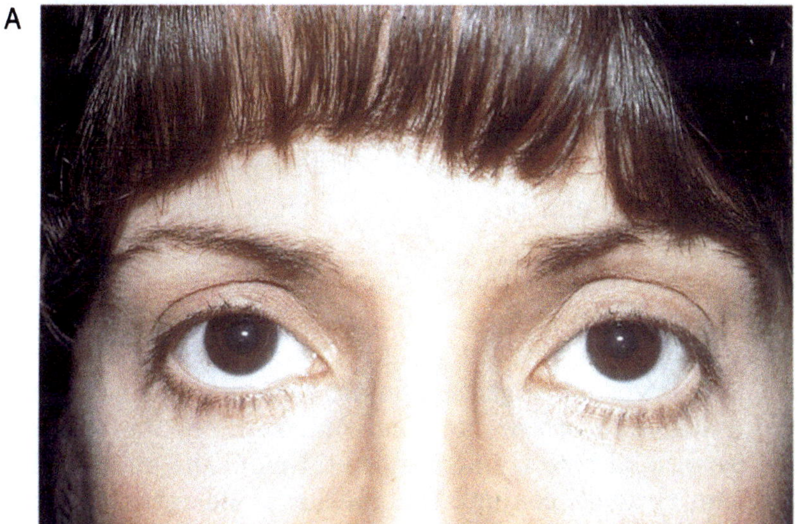

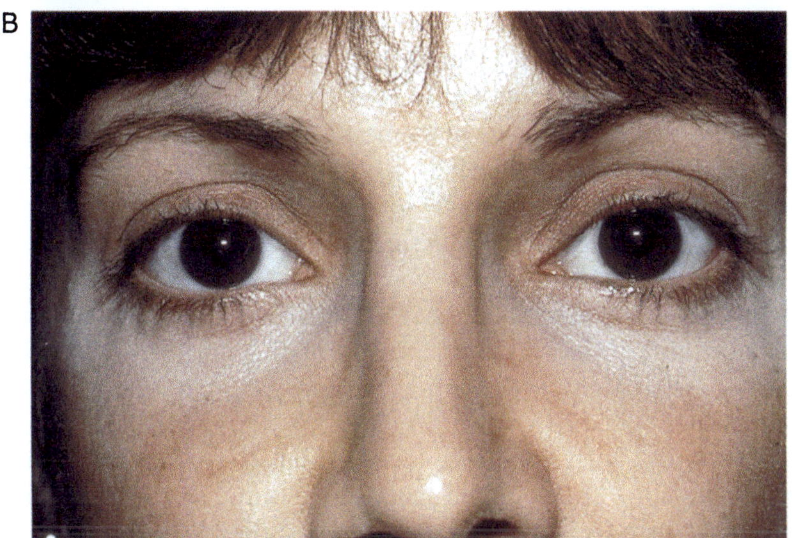

FIGURE 9.8. (A) Preoperative and (B) postoperative appearance of a patient with cicatricial lower eyelid retraction who underwent bilateral midface reconstruction. Augmentation of the anterior lamella obviated the need for a skin graft. The middle lamellar tether was splinted with an Alloderm graft.

COMPLICATIONS

Complications may occur at any step during this complex procedure. They are best avoided with a thorough knowledge of the underlying anatomy. It is sometimes possible to avoid reconstructive surgery altogether if physician and patient allow enough time for the middle lamellar tether to soften (a period of several months).

An excessively long canthotomy incision may create an obvious scar. This complication can be avoided by keeping the incision approximately 10 to 15 mm in length. Many patients with post-blepharoplasty lower lid retraction do not have significant horizontal laxity. To avoid inadvertent horizontal shortening, the cantholysis should be performed directly at the orbital rim. The subtarsal horizontal incision through conjunctiva and lower lid retractors should proceed medially to or through the caruncle to gain adequate exposure and elevation medially.

During the dissection toward the orbital rim, care should be taken to avoid piercing the fibrous septa, which hold back the orbital fat. Prolapsed orbital fat makes placement of the suspension sutures somewhat more difficult and risks a greater degree of postoperative scarring. If the fat does prolapse into the field, the surgeon should avoid purchasing the fat when placing the suspension sutures through the superior cuff of periosteum.

Bleeding is sometimes encountered in the area of the sutura notha upon incision and superior undermining of the periosteum. This can be controlled with light monopolar cautery or bone wax. The facial mimetic muscles are quite vascular, and bleeding under the flap can usually be avoided with adequate local infiltration of an epinephrine-containing solution. The solution frequently must be reinjected at approximately 45-minute intervals during the procedure to prevent diffuse oozing. If bleeding is encountered under the flap, it may be treated with light monopolar or bipolar cautery, although care must be taken to avoid injuring the overlying facial nerve.

Bleeding from the infraorbital neurovascular bundle can be avoided by cautious dissection in the area of the foramen. It is not uncommon to encounter some bleeding just superior to the foramen in the area of the origin of the levator labii superioris alaeque nasi muscle. This is a sign that the dissection is in close proximity to the infraorbital nerve, so the dissection must proceed carefully. Bleeding from the origin of this muscle may typically be controlled with light monopolar cautery with care to avoid the nerve. Cautery of the nerve may result in a painful postoperative neuroma, or hypesthesia in the distribution of the nerve.

The arcus marginalis should be incised approximately 2 mm inferior to the inferior orbital rim. This 2 mm cuff of periosteum, which will later be used to suspend the SOOF, tends to retract somewhat, so care must be taken to create enough tissue to allow for a good purchase with the cheek suspension sutures. If the cuff retracts and cannot be purchased, or if the periosteum is thin and attenuated from previous surgery, the surgeon may create 1 mm drill holes through the rim to allow for suspension sutures. Care must be taken to avoid purchasing the origin of the inferior oblique when the SOOF is suspended to the medial cuff of periosteum.

Inadequate medial elevation and augmentation may result in a suboptimal outcome. This can be avoided by thorough medial dissection and inferior periosteotomy. The surgeon can obtain improved medial exposure by continuing the horizontal incision to the caruncle.

The periosteotomy must begin sufficiently medially to obtain release and augmentation. The periosteotomy provides release of the SOOF to allow further cheek elevation. If the periosteotomy is inadequate, the cheek will not become mobile and may not be augmented properly. A curved periosteal elevator may be introduced under the flap to aid in the separation at the periosteal incision.

If the incision enters the buccal sulcus, the gingiva is repaired with several interrupted 5-0 mild chromic sutures toward the end of the procedure. Further dissection of the cheek can even be accomplished through the mouth, although this may increase the chance of postoperative infection, especially in patients with cheek or tear-trough implants.

Dimpling of the skin may result in areas overlying the SOOF suspension sutures. This complication can be avoided by checking for dimpling before and after placement of each suspension suture. If dimpling exists after placement of the suture, it must be cut and replaced with a deeper bite.

Postoperative hemorrhage may occur from any of the operated tissues. This uncommon complication can usually be avoided through meticulous intraoperative hemostasis and the use of a postoperative pressure dressing. If postoperative bleeding is encountered, the surgeon must first determine the location of the hemorrhage. If the hemorrhage is retrobulbar, emergent action must be undertaken, including aspiration, opening of the wound with evacuation, or even emergent orbital expansion to relieve a refractory compressive optic

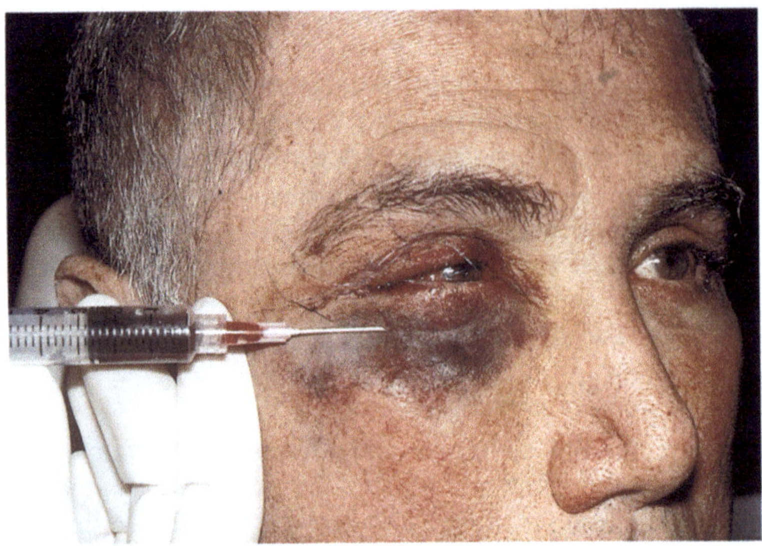

FIGURE 9.9. Treatment of acute postoperative hematoma. The patient experienced a severe bleeding episode approximately 12 hours following surgery. The hematoma was determined to be preseptal and was treated with ice packs and pressure. Over the following days, the organizing hematoma was aspirated to decrease the likelihood of postoperative middle lamellar cicatrix formation

neuropathy. Fortunately, the site of acute postoperative hemorrhage is frequently preseptal (Fig. 9.9). Bleeding of this nature may typically be controlled with ice packs and pressure. To minimize the chance of recurrent postoperative middle lamellar tether, the surgeon may aspirate or evacuate the organizing hematoma during the first several postoperative days.

Patients may be able to palpate nonabsorbable suture postoperatively through the thin tissues overlying the orbital rim. This may be avoided by cutting the Prolene sutures short, or by using absorbable suture, such as PDS.

Patients frequently are dissatisfied with asymmetric or low lateral canthal angles. This occurrence can be reduced by sitting the patient upright after temporary placement of the lateral tarsal suture. To tighten the angle and avoid rounding, a circular stitch of 6-0 mild chromic suture may be placed through the gray line in addition to a vertical mattress suture through skin and the gray line at the proposed angle.

    Subperiosteal Midface Lift

Many patients complain of postoperative discomfort. Occasionally, a patient may require removal of the Frost suture. Frequently, untoward postoperative pain is due to corneal abrasion by one of the posterior lamellar graft sutures. This situation can be avoided by burying all suture knots away from the cornea. The authors frequently place a bandage contact lens toward the end of the surgery and remove it approximately one week postoperatively, when the Frost suture is removed. The authors also reposition the Frost suture temporarily if the eye must be evaluated for postoperative pain.

10

ECTROPION

*Daniel E. Buerger

Ectropion is an outward rotation of the eyelid in which the lid margin is no longer in apposition to the globe. This situation results in exposure of the palpebral and bulbar conjunctiva as well as the cornea. Drying of the conjunctiva causes inflammation, which results in worsening of the condition and in chronic cases leads to keratinization of the conjunctival surface. The exposure may cause keratitis, chronic conjunctivitis, pain, photophobia, epiphora, and visual loss.[1]

Ectropion is generally classified by etiology into congenital, involutional, paralytic, cicatricial, inflammatory, and mechanical.[1] Most cases are involutional. Usually horizontal lid laxity is the primary etiological factor in involutional ectropion, but other factors often contribute to the condition. To minimize surgical failures and recurrences, all the etiological factors need to be recognized and treated appropriately.

EVALUATION

A careful examination of the patient's eyelids and face will reveal the cause of the ectropion as well as related conditions, such as eyelid retraction. Conditions that may affect the outcome of any surgical procedure, such as proptosis, enophthalmos, anophthalmos, or a flat malar eminence with descent of the midface, should be documented. This evaluation is by far the most important step in deciding the course of management.

During examination, patients with involutional ectropion will show some degree of eyelid laxity, which occurs as a result of tissue relaxation and the effects of gravity over time. Laxity is demonstrated by using the "snapback" test, in which the eyelid is gently pulled down and away from the globe. A normal lid quickly returns, or "snaps," back to its normal position, while a lax lid slowly drifts back toward the globe (Fig. 10.1). Sometimes a blink is required before the lid returns to complete apposition to the globe,[2] indicating moderate to severe laxity.

The "pinch" test (or "distraction" test), in which the eyelid is pulled away from the globe, is another test for eyelid laxity.[3] A forward displacement of 6 to 8 mm or more is abnormal, demonstrating that the lid is lax. In practice, the snapback test usually suffices to demonstrate horizontal laxity, and the pinch test is rarely necessary.

Lateral canthal tendon laxity is tested by pulling the lid medially. If the horizontal distance between the canthal angle and the temporal limbus is shortened, then laxity of the lateral canthal tendon is present.[3] Rounding of the lateral canthal angle and several millimeters of thinning of the lateral lower lid margin are also signs of lateral canthal tendon laxity.

The surgeon must also consider the possibility of laxity or disinsertion of the lower lid retractors. This possibility is usually considered in the context of entropion, but it can play an important role in ectropion as well. Repairing laxity of the lower lid retractors helps to stabilize a floppy tarsus.

Medial canthal tendon laxity is tested by pulling the eyelid laterally. If the punctum is displaced laterally 6 to 8 mm toward the nasal limbus, then significant medial canthal tendon laxity is present. If this factor is missed or ignored when horizontally shortening the lid, the punctum will be permanently displaced laterally[3] and punctal eversion may persist afterward.

Cicatricial changes to the anterior lamella must also be evaluated. A lower lid that has been everted for many months may develop cicatrization and shortening of the anterior lamella. Once this has occurred, routine correction of ectropion will not be effective.[3] Other causes of cicatricial ectropion are thermal or chemical burns, mechanical or surgical trauma, and secondary contraction from chronic inflammation such as seen with acne rosacea, dermatitis, and ic-

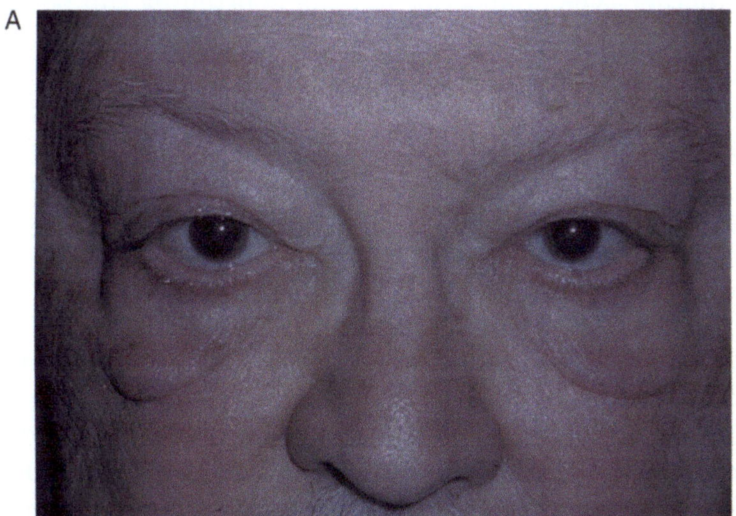

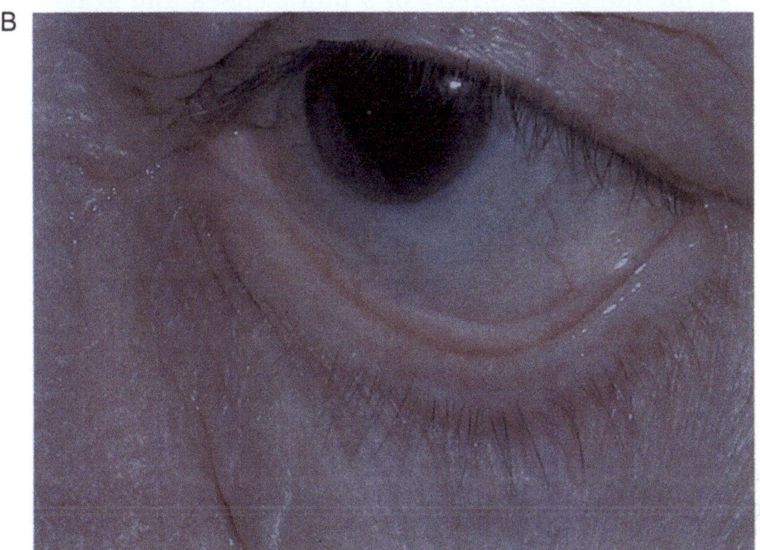

FIGURE 10.1. "Snapback" test involves pulling the lower lid away from the globe. (A) Patient with festoons and inferior scleral show (B) After release in this patient, the lid does not return to its normal position, suggesting the presence of severe laxity.

thyosis. Another type of anterior lamella shortening can be found in patients with severe descent of the midface pulling on the lower eyelid, especially in patients with a flat malar eminence.

Examination for cicatricial changes is performed by pulling the lid superiorly. If the margin does not reach 2 mm above the inferior limbers, the lid is vertically deficient.[3] Another method to determine the adequacy of the anterior lamella is to have the patient look up and open the mouth. Shortening of the anterior lamella will be evident as the lid pulls down when the mouth is opened. If the anterior lamella is shortened with cicatricial changes, it must be lengthened with insertion of a skin graft or a Z-plasty at the time of horizontal shortening.

In paralytic ectropion resulting from dysfunction of the facial (seventh cranial) nerve, the canthal tendons are frequently normal. However, loss of orbicularis muscle tone results in outward displacement of the lower lid due to the effects of a ptotic cheek and gravity.[2] With a long-standing paralytic eyelid, the downward forces stretch the canthal tendons (Fig. 10.2).

Mechanical ectropion is usually caused by bulky tumors of the eyelids or conjunctiva and is usually easily diagnosed. Less obvious

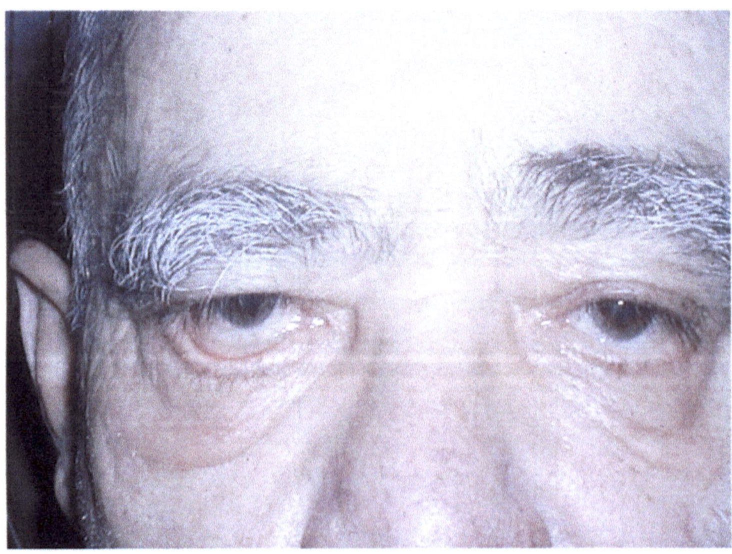

FIGURE 10.2. Paralytic ectropion.

causes include fluid accumulations, herniated orbital fat, anophthalmos with a heavy ocular prosthesis, or poorly fitted spectacles. Treatment involves medical or surgical elimination of the causative factors.

When a careful preoperative assessment is complete and an understanding of the anatomical changes is present, the course of therapy can be decided. There are numerous procedures or combinations of procedures from which to choose, and the surgeon should realize that none is effective in every instance.[1] Treatment must be individualized to correct the deficiencies found during the examination of that particular patient.

TECHNIQUE

Horizontal Shortening of the Lower Eyelid: The Lateral Tarsal Strip Procedure

Horizontal shortening of the eyelid by the lateral tarsal strip procedure is one of the most commonly performed procedures in ophthalmic plastic surgery. It is useful in the repair of ectropion when there is mild to moderate horizontal laxity of the eyelid, which is usually secondary to involutional changes with stretching of the lateral canthal tendon or the entire tarsoligamentous sling. The lateral canthal tendon is thinner and weaker than the medial canthal tendon, and in involutional cases is usually the first to become lax. When medial canthal tendon laxity is present, it should also be addressed surgically.

The most important pitfalls with this surgery, especially for beginning surgeons, are inaccurate placement of the sutures to reattach the tarsus to the orbital rim and improper tightening of the lid. Proper placement of the sutures is the key to avoiding lateral canthal angle dystopia and poor apposition of the eyelid to the globe. The lid must be reattached high enough (superiorly) and internal enough (posteriorly) to give a proper inward and upward contour to the lower eyelid.[4] Normally, the lateral canthal tendon is attached 1 to 2 mm higher than the medial canthal tendon and is attached just inside the lateral orbital rim at the lateral orbital tubercle.

In the performance of the lateral canthotomy, adequate exposure of the lateral orbital rim will help facilitate placement of the sutures. This is best accomplished by cutting all the way down to the lateral

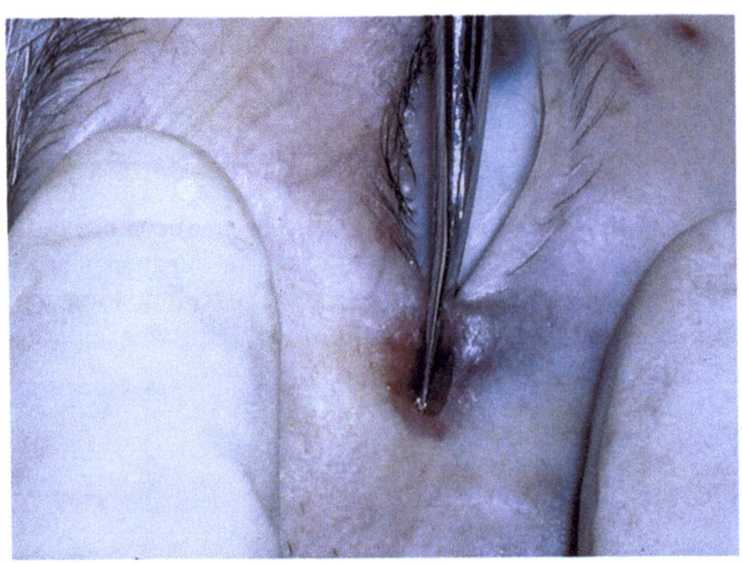

FIGURE 10.3. Lateral canthotomy incision is extended to the periosteum.

orbital rim periosteum with the initial canthotomy incision (Fig. 10.3). Frequently, the orbicularis over the rim is difficult to remove with scissors, and adequate visualization of the periosteum is achieved by incising with cautery.[5]

There are numerous methods to create a tarsal strip, all of which involve removing the skin, orbicularis, and conjunctiva surrounding the end of the tarsus. For a surgeon without an assistant, a few points may facilitate handling and development of the strip. Many surgeons perform an inferior cantholysis first and free the lower part of the tarsus. However, this step makes the tarsus more mobile. If the maneuver is saved for later, the tarsus remains less mobile, and removal of the surrounding tissue is easier.

The tarsus can be stabilized by pulling laterally and superiorly. The extent of tissue removal depends on the amount of eyelid laxity and planned tarsal shortening. With Westcott scissors, several millimeters of anterior lamella are easily removed. The eyelid (superior) margin can also be removed with scissors or a blade. The posterior aspect (conjunctiva) is debrided with a blade. Inferior cantholysis is

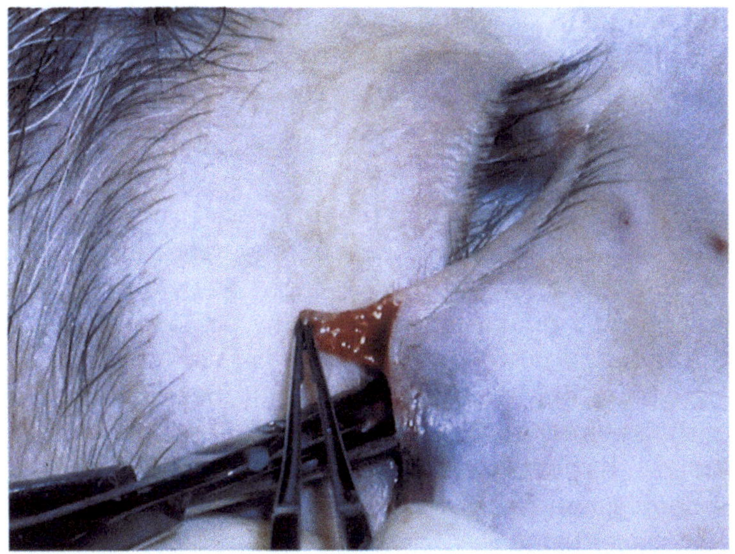

FIGURE 10.4. Inferior cantholysis may be performed before or after tarsal strip is created. Intraoperative photograph demonstrates inferior cantholysis and lysing of middle lamellar scar tissue, following formation of an adequate tarsal strip.

then completed with scissors; middle lamellar scarring may also be incised through the canthal incision (Fig. 10.4). The lower eyelid should be mobile.

The tarsal strip is pulled laterally to mimic its final position. Excess tarsus that overlaps the rim (usually 2–3 mm) should be removed. A mattress suture is used to secure the end of the tarsus to the periosteum of the inner aspect of the lateral orbital rim.

During placement of the sutures, small half-circle needles are passed through the periosteum just inside the lateral orbital rim, about 1 mm higher than the normal canthal tendon attachment. To help visualize the rim during suture placement, a cotton-tipped applicator is placed just inside the rim and pushed posteriorly. This maneuver isolates the rim from the surrounding tissues and allows for good suture placement. Two bites are passed through the lateral tarsus and orbital rim, either as interrupted sutures or in a horizontal mattress fashion. The sutures are placed about 2 mm apart. When the sutures are tied, the lid should be firmly against the globe and the lid should rest about 1 to 2 mm higher than the medial canthal tendon, as shown earlier (see Fig. 9.7). The position of the eyelid height can be adjusted by varying the suture tension. If the lid is placed too high or too low, or if it is not in apposition to the globe laterally, the sutures should be removed and replaced to correct the problem.

It is important to emphasize that proper placement of the tarsal sutures intraoperatively avoids the postoperative complications of lateral canthal angle dystopia. The inexperienced surgeon often places the angle too low (below the orbital tubercle), resulting in inferior displacement of the lateral canthus.[1] A slight elevation is tolerable because there is some relaxation and sagging postoperatively. Massaging the canthal angle postoperatively may help lower the angle a small amount. Excessive elevation is sometimes difficult to detect with the patient in the supine position and may not be noticeable until the patient is upright. Patients tend to notice an elevation of the angle more so than a depression. Excessive elevation often resolves, and seldom needs to be repositioned.

COMPLICATIONS

There are two main reasons for failure of the lateral tarsal strip procedure. Persistence or undercorrection of the laxity occurs frequently because of failure to adequately shorten the lid. With the patient in a supine position, the laxity is less obvious because the effects of gravity are not present. As the sutures at the lateral orbital rim are tied, the tension on the lid can be adjusted by tightening the suture. If the eyelid is drawn too tightly, it may appear to slide inferiorly under the curvature of the globe.[5] It is best to slightly overtighten the lid intraoperatively because some relaxation or stretching will occur over the first few weeks postoperatively.

The other reason for persistent laxity postoperatively is failure to secure the tarsus to the periosteum laterally. If the suture is not passed through the periosteum, it will not adequately support the lid postoperatively. This may result in rounding of the canthal angle, and later, recurrence of the ectropion. Adequate exposure of the lateral orbital rim, as described earlier, allows for easier and more accurate placement of the sutures. To ensure that a good bite of periosteum is present, the surgeon should grab both sides of the suture after it has been placed and pull away from the rim. If good support is present, the suture will feel tight and remain immobile.

Excessive tightening of the eyelid or overcorrection is a rare problem postoperatively because the lid will stretch over several weeks.

Intraoperatively, it may occur if the tarsal strip is cut too short prior to suture placement. If this occurs, a small periosteal flap may be created at the lateral orbital rim and may be secured to the tarsus. One can avoid this problem by excising the excess tarsus only after the sutures have been secured to the orbital rim.

Excessive tightening is a more serious problem when other anatomical changes are present but not initially appreciated. Patients with prominent globes, secondary to either shallow orbits or high myopia and long axial length, or patients with proptosis, should be approached with caution. Even mild overtightening in these patients will cause the eyelid to slide under the globe and give the appearance of eyelid retraction.

Patients who have a flat malar eminence also require special attention (Fig. 10.5). Preoperatively they manifest significant horizontal laxity because the chronic pull of the cheek loosens the lateral canthal tendon. In a supine position, the lack of facial support from the underlying bones is not evident. When the patient is upright, more vertical traction is present, which sets up a predisposition to an early recurrence of laxity and potentially ectropion.

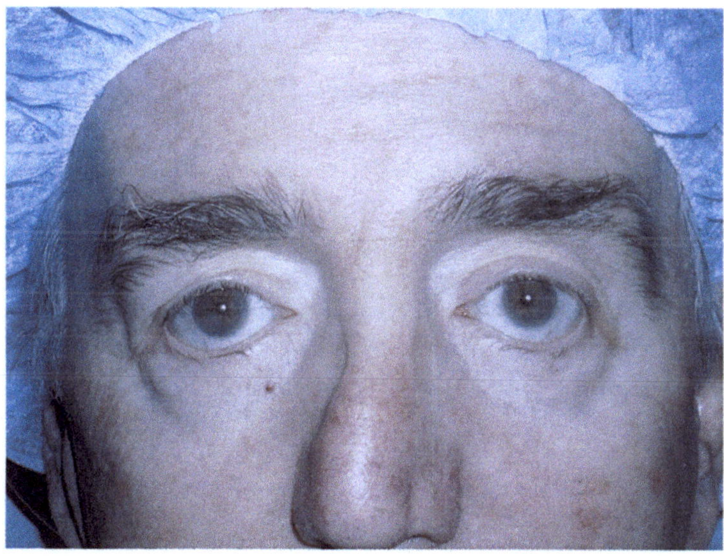

FIGURE 10.5. Patients with flat malar eminence and lower eyelid retraction are predisposed to an early recurrence of eyelid malposition.

Other complications of the lateral tarsal strip procedure usually do not cause recurrent ectropion but can be irritating to the patient. Trichiasis at the lateral canthus results from a failure to excise the excess lash-bearing marginal skin that is pulled beyond the canthal angle during the shortening of the lid. These lashes, if irritating to the patient, can be epilated or removed by electrocautery.

Conjunctival cysts can occur postoperatively if the tarsal strip is not de-epithelialized of conjunctiva prior to suture placement. Residual epithelial cells can be buried, resulting in cyst formation. Scraping the tarsal strip with a #15 Bard–Parker blade will remove the conjunctival epithelium.

Redundancy of the lateral eyelid skin may be seen if significant shortening of the lid is performed without excision of the anterior lamella, skin, and orbicularis. Preoperative dermatochalasis of the lower lid contributes to the problem. When this situation is noted preoperatively or intraoperatively, a subciliary incision may be extended several millimeters medially across the lid. The excess anterior lamella is then draped over the wound laterally and excised in the same manner as an external lower blepharoplasty.

TECHNIQUES

Lateral Canthal Tendon Plication

The lateral canthal tendon plication is useful when there is mild horizontal laxity causing ectropion. This procedure is very useful for mild degrees of laxity; however, when involutional ectropion develops, there is usually at least moderate horizontal laxity. A suture plication alone is rarely adequate to provide long-term ectropion repair.

A benefit of this procedure is that it minimizes the risks of lateral canthal angle dystopia. As with the lateral tarsal strip procedure, suture placement is the key to a successful outcome. The medial aspect of the common crus may be plicated to its lateral projection, or preferably to the periosteum of the lateral orbital rim (Fig. 10.6). Care must be taken to place the sutures through the periosteum of the lateral orbital rim at the same position as the attachments of the canthal tendon or slightly superiorly. Alternatively, the inferior crus (or lateral aspect of tarsus) may be plicated to the periosteum, as shown earlier (see Fig. 2.6). This maneuver may accomplish mild elevation of the lower lid. Some surgeons advocate lateral canthopexy

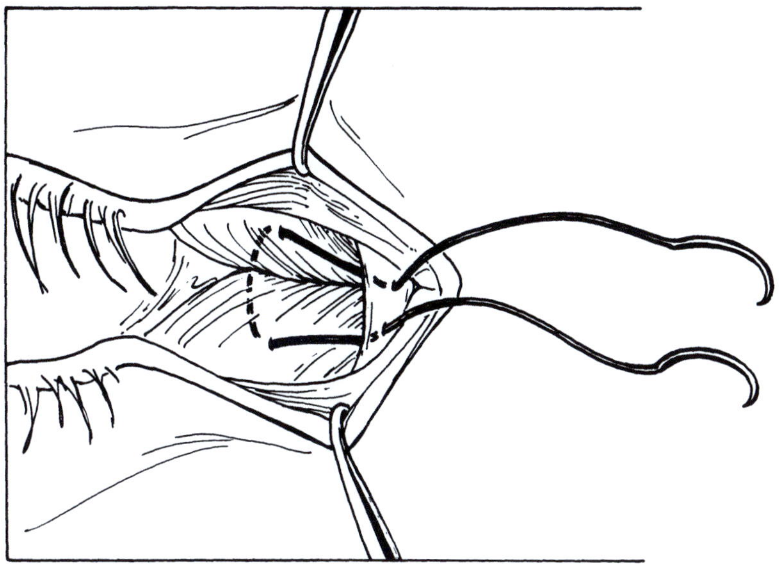

FIGURE 10.6. Lateral canthal tendon plication, with placement of the suture to secure the common crus of the lateral canthal tendon to the orbital rim. (Reproduced with permission from Classification and treatment of eyelid malposition. In: Nesi FA, Gladstone GJ, Brazzo BG, et al, eds. *Ophthalmic and Facial Plastic Surgery: A Compendium of Reconstructive and Aesthetic Techniques*. Thorofare, NJ: Slack Incorporated; 2000:94.)

(plication) through a small canthal or upper blepharoplasty incision (see Chapter 8).

Medial Canthal Tendon Plication

When medial canthal tendon laxity is present and contributing to the horizontal laxity and ectropion formation, the medial canthal tendon needs to be repaired. Performing an isolated lateral procedure will cause displacement of the lacrimal punctum and dysfunction of the lacrimal drainage system.

There are several methods of medial canthal tendon plication. The anterior approach through the skin provides better visualization of the canthal tendon for suture placement. The anterior approach plicates the anterior limb of the canthal tendon; however, the posterior limb is responsible for keeping the eyelid in apposition to the globe. When medial canthal tendon laxity is a contributing factor to ectro-

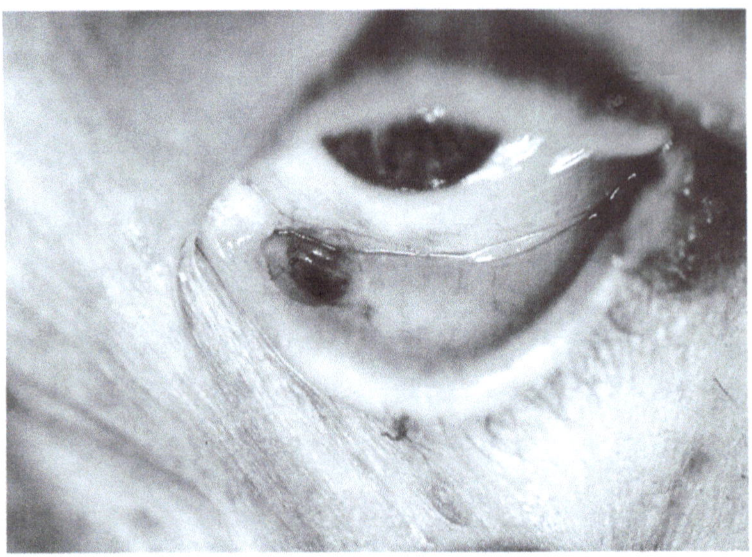

FIGURE 10.7. Diamond-shaped excision of conjunctiva and lower lid retractors inferior to the lacrimal punctum.

pion, there is some degree of laxity of the posterior limb. For this reason, correction via the posterior (transconjunctival) approach is the more anatomically correct procedure.

In this procedure, a diamond-shaped wedge of conjunctiva and retractors (approximately 6 mm horizontally and 4 mm vertically) is removed (Fig. 10.7). By means of blunt dissection with Westcott scissors, the surgeon develops a tunnel toward the posterior lacrimal crest. Dissection proceeds approximately 10 mm, until the bony crest is reached.

A double-armed 5-0 Prolene suture with small OPS needles is used for fixation. Both ends of the suture are passed through the inferomedial corner of the exposed tarsus. Fine forceps are passed into the previously formed tunnel to the posterior lacrimal crest, and a small amount of tissue corresponding to the medial aspect of the medial canthal tendon is gently pulled through the conjunctival tunnel. This deep tissue is tied to the inferomedial tarsus by passing the sutures from lateral to medial (anterior to posterior), completing the mattress

                                                                    Ectropion

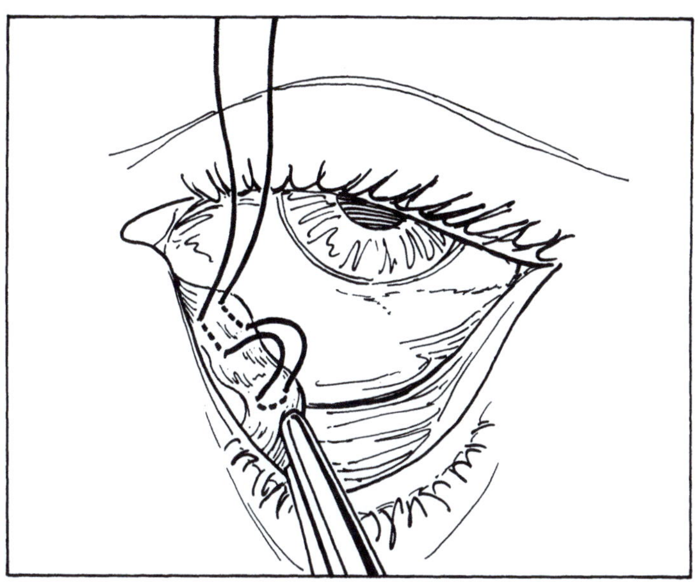

FIGURE 10.8. Medial canthal plication, with a mattress suture securing the medial tarsus to the posterior limb of the medial canthal tendon. (Reproduced with permission from Classification and treatment of eyelid malposition. In: Nesi FA, Gladstone GJ, Brazzo BG, et al, eds. *Ophthalmic and Facial Plastic Surgery: A Compendium of Reconstructive and Aesthetic Techniques.* Thorofare, NJ: Slack Incorporated; 2000:96.)

stitch (Fig. 10.8). The conjunctiva is closed with several vertical interrupted 6-0 plain gut sutures.

When the plication suture is secure, the punctum will move into appropriate horizontal position and assume a tighter position. The punctum will become posteriorly displaced so that it is in apposition to the globe. Conjunctival closure may assist in rotating the punctum inward.

COMPLICATIONS

Regardless of the approach used, the complications of medial canthal plication are similar. As with lateral canthal tendon plication, it is difficult to cause canthal angle dystopia with plication sutures, and particular attention to proper suture placement will reduce any chances of this occurring. Placing the sutures slightly superior to the normal anatomical attachments helps support the lid and takes into account the loosening of the lid postoperatively.

The major complication with medial canthal tendon plication sutures is canalicular occlusion. Certainly any suture passed through the canaliculus can occlude its lumen or cause enough scarring to produce canalicular strictures, possibly resulting in epiphora. Placing a Bowman probe in the canaliculus during the procedure will help identify the course of the canaliculus so that it can be avoided during suture placement.

Even without disrupting the canaliculus with the sutures, epiphora can result from a buckling of the canaliculus as the sutures are tightened. The surgeon should avoid trying to accomplish too much with this procedure. Horizontal laxity rarely results from medial canthal tendon laxity alone, so the surgeon should not try to correct the horizontal laxity with only medial canthal tendon plication. This procedure is used to stabilize the medial canthal tendon only.

Medial Spindle Procedure

Punctal eversion with or without medial ectropion is addressed with the medial spindle procedure. The medial spindle procedure is a resection of conjunctiva and lower lid retractors in an elliptical or diamond shape, approximately 6 to 8 mm horizontally and 3 to 5 mm vertically. The ellipse is centered about 4 mm below the punctum (see Fig. 10.7). For the mild cases, the edges of the wound may be simply closed with an absorbable suture. To achieve a more significant correction, the sutures are passed full thickness through the lid, aiming down through the inferior fornix, to a point 10 to 12 mm below the lid margin, and tied on the skin over a bolster (Fig. 10.9).

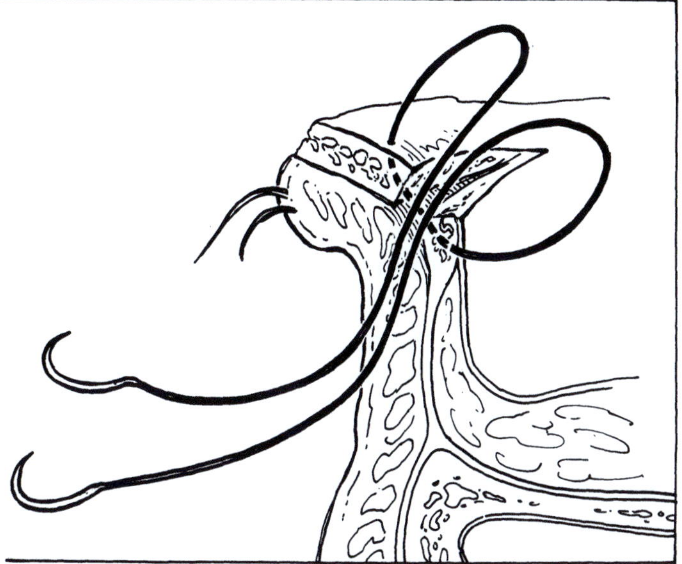

FIGURE 10.9. Medial spindle procedure. Suture placement through full-thickness eyelid to aid in inward rotation. (Reproduced with permission from Classification and treatment of eyelid malposition. In: Nesi FA, Gladstone GJ, Brazzo BG, et al, eds. *Ophthalmic and Facial Plastic Surgery: A Compendium of Reconstructive and Aesthetic Techniques.* Thorofare, NJ: Slack Incorporated; 2000:100.)

Complications

The main complications of this procedure are recurrence of the ectropion and canalicular injury. In terms of recurrence, this procedure is usually not sufficient on its own to correct a full-eyelid ectropion. Most patients who have punctal ectropion also have full-eyelid ectropion, or at least have significant eyelid retraction or laxity. Therefore, the spindle procedure is often used in conjunction with some type of lid-shortening procedure. If medial canthal tendon laxity is also present, consideration should be given to plicating the tendon. The plication can be performed through the same incision as the spindle procedure, and closure of the wound will assist in inverting the punctum.

Canalicular injury results from placing the excision too high (superiorly) on the conjunctival surface or from poor suture placement.

Placing a Bowman probe in the lower canaliculus at the beginning of
the procedure not only helps to prevent this problem, but also can aid
in the exposure of the inferior fornix during the surgery.

CICATRICIAL ECTROPION REPAIR

Vertical shortening of the anterior lamella results in a cicatricial ectropion (Fig. 10.10). There are multiple potential causes of cicatricial
changes to the anterior lamella as mentioned earlier. The cicatrix may
involve skin, subcutaneous tissue, orbicularis, and/or septum. Detecting the proper location of the cicatrix is essential for proper surgical planning.

When the cicatricial changes result from trauma or surgery, digital massage is often recommended to help soften and stretch the scar.
This can be done in combination with steroid injections, 0.1 to 0.2 mL
of triamcinolone (10–25 mg/mL) directly into the area of cicatrix. Injections may be performed two to three times, at least a week apart,
and are most effective if instituted within 6 weeks of the acute event.

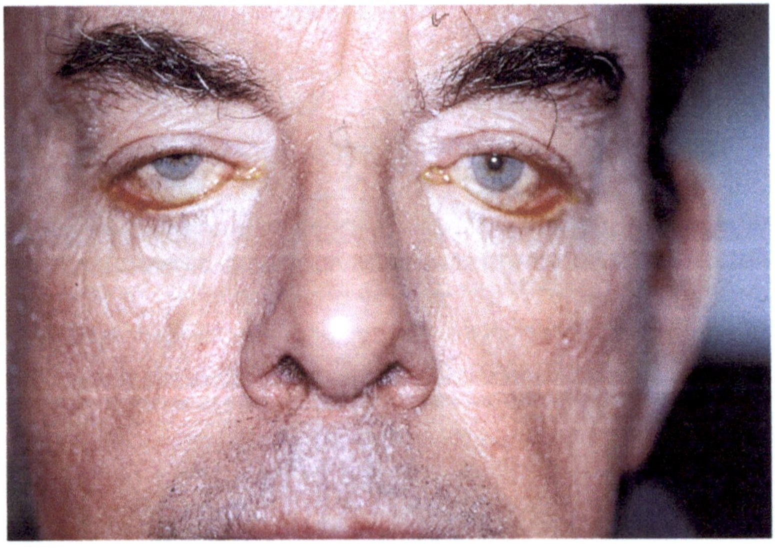

FIGURE 10.10. Bilateral lower eyelid cicatricial ectropion with
icthyosis.

Unless there are signs of severe exposure, it is best to wait at least
6 months prior to any surgical repair to allow the scar to soften. If
severe exposure develops, a suture tarsorrhaphy can be placed to give
the scar time to soften.

If the cicatricial changes are isolated to one area of the eyelid, either a small full-thickness wedge resection or a Z-plasty with excision of subcutaneous scar tissue can be performed. For larger areas
of scarring or skin deficit, a skin graft is usually required. If there is
associated horizontal laxity, this situation must be corrected at the
same time.

When one is performing a skin graft to repair a cicatricial ectropion, a full-thickness skin graft is preferable to a split-thickness graft.
A full-thickness graft gives a better match to the surrounding tissues
and has less postoperative contraction. Full-thickness grafts that give
the best match in terms of color and thickness to eyelid skin can be
harvested from the upper eyelids (Fig. 10.11), the retroauricular or
supraclavicular area, or the inner aspect of the upper arm.

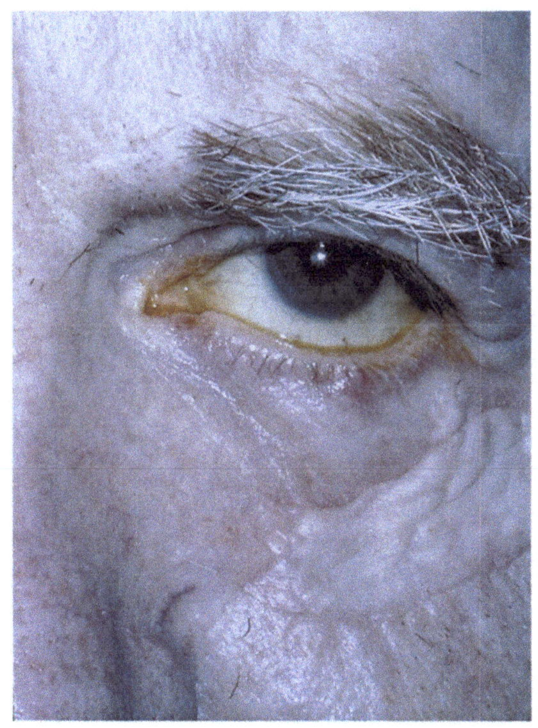

FIGURE 10.11. Healed skin
graft on the left lower eyelid after repair of cicatricial ectropion
(different patient from Fig.
10.10). The full-thickness skin
graft was taken from the supraclavicular area. Patient has
moderate graft contracture with
lower lid retraction.

Complications

Complications of cicatricial ectropion repair generally fall into two categories: persistent or recurrent ectropion, and graft failure. As with all procedures, attention to proper surgical technique will minimize these risks.

Persistent or recurrent ectropion is usually caused by a failure to completely release the cicatricial bands. The proper level of the cicatricial contracture (skin, muscle, or septum) must be determined so that it can be released. Detection and removal of scar tissue are facilitated if the cicatrix is placed on tension.[5] One or two 4-0 silk traction sutures are placed through the lid margin to keep the lid on stretch during the procedure. The cicatricial bands can be palpated, and all areas must be released. An endpoint to cicatricial band lysis is good mobility of the lid, and for lower eyelids this means having the ability to pull the lid over the pupil without localized tension.

Another cause of recurrent ectropion is failure to account for graft contracture (Fig. 10.11). Full-thickness grafts will contract, or shrink, less than split-thickness grafts. Even with full-thickness grafts (Fig. 10.12), the surgeon must account for some contracture postoperatively. Before measuring for the graft size, the eyelid must be placed on stretch to get an accurate determination of graft size. A good rule is that the graft should be 1.5 times the width of the shortest vertical dimension of the recipient defect.[2] The lid must be left on stretch with traction, using either a suture tarsorrhaphy or a Frost-type suture from the lower eyelid to the brow area, for the first 7 to 10 days postoperatively.

Graft failure is unusual owing to the rich vascularity of the eyelids and the thinness of the graft. Early, if the graft appears dark colored and failure is suspected, debridement should be resisted. Frequently the viable lower dermis will eventually reepithelialize if left undisturbed for a week prior to any debridement.[4]

For the graft to survive, it must stay in apposition to the recipient bed so that the new blood supply can reach the graft. A bolster or good pressure dressing should support the graft against its bed for 4 to 5 days. Hematoma formation, which elevates the graft away from its blood supply, is one of the most common problems that results in graft failure. Adequate hemostasis of the recipient bed is necessary to prevent the possibility of hematoma formation. The surgeon should be careful not to use overly aggressive cautery either, because the vascular supply can be compromised if a layer of char debris deposits

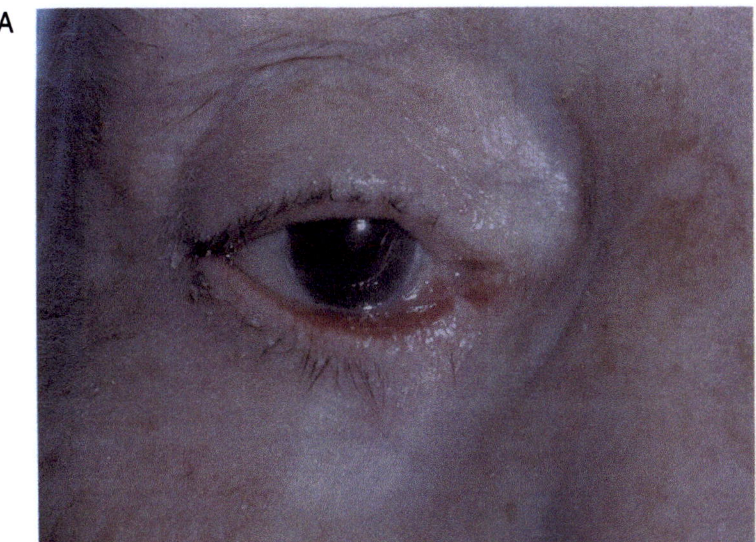

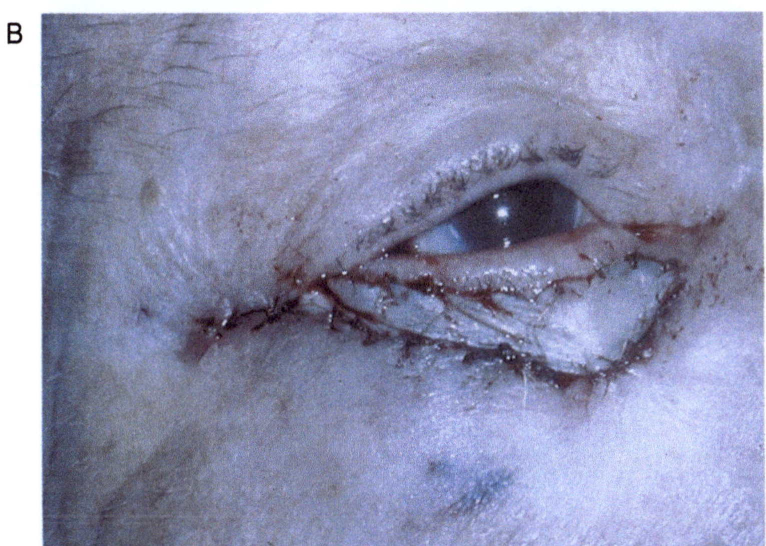

FIGURE 10.12. (A) Patient with severe right lower eyelid cicatricial ectropion, following cryotherapy of basal cell carcinoma. (B) Immediate postoperative view of retroauricular skin graft following lysis of cicatrix and lateral tarsal strip procedure.

between the recipient bed and the graft. The placement of numerous fenestrations through the graft allows for drainage of fluid and helps to prevent graft contracture.

REFERENCES

1. Paris GL, Garber PF. Classification and correction of ectropion. In: Stewart WB, ed. *Surgery of the Eyelid, Orbit, and Lacrimal System*. Vol 2. *Ophthalmology Monographs* 8. San Francisco: American Academy of Ophthalmology; 1994:53–83.

2. Dutton JJ. Ectropion. In: Dutton JJ, ed. *Atlas of Ophthalmic Surgery*. Vol II. *Oculoplastic, Lacrimal, and Orbital Surgery*. St. Louis: Mosby-Year Book; 1992:94–113.

3. Bosniak SL, Zilkha MC. Ectropion. In: Nesi FA, Lisman RD, Levine MR, eds. *Smith's Ophthalmic Plastic and Reconstructive Surgery*. 2d ed. St Louis: Mosby-Year Book; 1998:290–307.

4. Wesley RE. Ectropion repair. In: McCord CD Jr, Tannenbaum M, Nunery WR, eds. *Oculoplastic Surgery*. 3rd ed. New York: Raven Press; 1995:249–261.

5. Classification and treatment of eyelid malposition. In Nesi FA, Gladstone GJ, Brazzo BG, et al, eds. *Ophthalmic and Facial Plastic Surgery: A Compendium of Reconstructive and Aesthetic Techniques*. Thorofare, NJ: Slack Incorporated; 2000:89–100.

11

ENTROPION

- Cassandra B. Onofrey
- David T. Tse

Involutional entropion is a common eyelid malposition that can lead to significant corneal epithelial disruption. Entropion may be precipitated by intraocular surgery or by other factors, resulting in a vicious cycle of ocular irritation, reflexive blepharospasm, and inward rotation of the eyelid margin. The resultant mechanical irritation further exacerbates the eyelid malposition problem. Such a scenario is referred to as spastic entropion, which is a variant of involutional entropion. Occasionally, entropion may become manifest without a precipitating event.[1]

The pathophysiology of involutional entropion (Fig. 11.1) has been well described.[1-20] Horizontal eyelid laxity[9-13] and lower eyelid retractors disinsertion/attenuation[2,3,11-20] lead to instability of the lower eyelid, manifesting in either entropion or ectropion depending on the net rotational force. Poor adhesion of the skin and pretarsal orbicularis to the tarsus can result in overriding of the preseptal orbicularis onto the pretarsal orbicularis with an inward rotation of the eyelid margin during eyelid closure.[2,3,7,8,15,19] Prolapse of the normal anteriorly protruding orbital fat within the lower eyelid was advanced as another pathogenic mechanism of involutional entropion, seen more frequently among Asians.[21]

Age-related orbital fat atrophy could produce involutional enophthalmos, which may destabilize the lid when the globe is not in firm apposition to the inner eyelid.[9] However, some authors doubt the importance of relative enophthalmos in the pathogenesis of entropion.[22] While there are compelling reasons to accept the current etiological hypotheses of involutional entropion, these are not proven, and they warrant further studies.

Many diseases can lead to vertical contracture of the posterior lamella of the eyelid, resulting in cicatricial entropion. Autoimmune

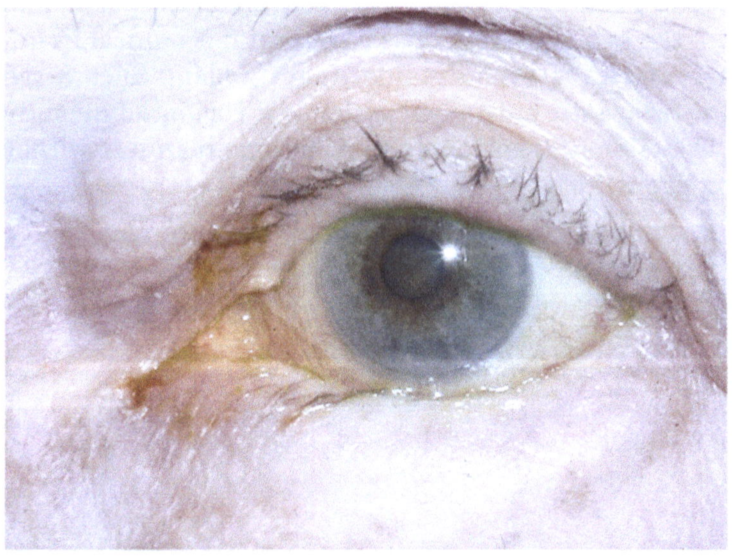

FIGURE 11.1. Lower eyelid entropion secondary to horizontal laxity and dehiscence of retractor muscles.

conditions (e.g., cicatricial pemphigoid), inflammatory diseases (e.g., Stevens–Johnson syndrome), infections (e.g., trachoma, herpes zoster), and chemical and thermal burns can all result in cicatricial changes.

Corneal and conjunctival abrasions are common in entropion because the lashes and skin constantly rub against the ocular surface. Patients usually complain of a chronic foreign body sensation, redness, tearing, and discharge. If uncorrected, this constant irritation can lead to secondary stromal scarring, corneal thinning, and vascularization. Corneal ulceration and perforation may occur in extreme cases.

EYELID ANATOMY

A thorough understanding of lower eyelid anatomy and function is essential for the evaluation and repair of entropion. The lower eyelid retractors are also referred to as the capsulopalpebral fascia. They are analogous to the levator aponeurosis and Muller's muscle of the upper eyelid. The capsulopalpebral fascia originates as the capsulopalpebral head with delicate attachments to the inferior rectus muscle and tendon. The capsulopalpebral head divides into two portions as it extends around and fuses with the sheath of the inferior oblique muscle. Anterior to the inferior oblique muscle, the two layers rejoin to form Lockwood's ligament. Anterior to Lockwood's ligament, the fascial tissue is termed the capsulopalpebral fascia.

A large portion of the capsulopalpebral fascia proceeds anteriorly to insert on the inferior fornix and to form Tenon's capsule on the globe. The main body of the fascia ascends the eyelid to insert onto the inferior margin of the tarsal plate. Dehiscence or disinsertion of the retractor attachments may render tarsus unstable, resulting in inward rotation of the lid margin. This is probably the most frequently encountered anatomical defect, yet it is the most difficult component of involutional entropion to detect clinically.

The lower eyelid retractors have fine extensions to the overlying orbicularis muscle and skin. A weakening of the extensions, along with loss of the attachments between the preseptal orbicularis muscle and the orbital septum, allows the preseptal orbicularis to override the pretarsal orbicularis. An acute inflammatory episode may also cause spasms of the orbicularis and precipitate temporary entropion. Today, most cases originally considered spastic actually represent involutional entropion with the typical lower eyelid pathology.

The lateral and medial canthal tendons rigidly anchor the lids to the orbital periosteum. With stretching of the lateral canthal tendon, lid changes such as horizontal laxity, displacement, and loss of elasticity occur. These changes may manifest either as entropion or ectropion, depending on the differential vector forces between the anterior and posterior lamellae of the lower lid.

EVALUATION

Horizontal eyelid laxity is primarily caused by dehiscence or stretching of the lateral canthal tendon. Lower eyelid tension can be assessed by pulling the central portion of the eyelid away from the globe ("pinch" or "distraction" test). If the lower eyelid can be distracted more than 6 to 8 mm from the globe, horizontal laxity is present. Pulling the lower eyelid inferiorly and then releasing it is a better method of assessing tension ("snapback" test described in Chapter 10: see Fig. 10.1). Upon release, a normal eyelid should snap back against the globe immediately. A severely lax eyelid may require one or more blinks to return to normal position.

In patients with lower eyelid retractor disinsertion or dehiscence, four clinical clues may be present. These clinical clues are similar to those associated with ectropion. First, the inferior fornix is deeper than that of the uninvolved eyelid. Anatomically, the capsulopalpebral fascia sends attachments to the inferior fornix, and when the retractors are disinserted, the inferior fornix is pulled inward. This situation results in a fornix that appears deeper. Second, the lower eyelid assumes a higher resting level when the involved eyelid is pulled out of its entropic position. This is because the retractors are no longer attached to the inferior margin of the tarsal plate, thus yielding to an unopposed orbicularis muscle that pulls the eyelid to a higher resting position. Third, a diminished lower eyelid excursion on downgaze is noted, owing to absence of attachment of the retractors to the tarsal plate. Fourth, the leading edge of the detached capsulopalpebral fascia may be visualized adjacent to a transverse red band below the inferior tarsal border. This red band is thought to be the orbicularis muscle fibers showing through the zone of retractor disinsertion.

Overriding of the preseptal orbicularis onto the pretarsal orbicularis may reproduce an intermittent entropion, which can be demonstrated by having the patient forcefully squeeze the eyelids. Occasionally, the examiner may need to recline the examination chair or place the patient in a recumbent position to uncover the entropion more easily.

Cicatricial entropion should be suspected if resistance to downward traction or outward rotation is present, or if horizontal traction on the lid does not temporarily improve the eyelid position. Fornix symblepharon may render the eyelid difficult to evert. The conjunctiva, lid margin, and meibomian glands should be inspected for conjunctival metaplasia and lash distortion.

Techniques

Numerous surgical procedures have been described to correct involutional entropion. The large number of distinct procedures attests to the multifactorial nature of the pathogenesis of involutional entropion and to the failure of any one technique to be entirely satisfactory. The surgical approach is aimed at correcting the underlying pathogenic mechanisms: horizontal eyelid laxity, retractor laxity/disinsertion, and vertical overriding of the preseptal orbicularis muscle. While correction of a single pathogenic factor may prove successful in some patients who have one predominant component responsible for the malposition, most experts suggest that correction of at least two of these three elements confers a greater chance for long-term success.

Full-Thickness Eyelid Sutures

Full-thickness eyelid sutures remain a popular office or bedside procedure for involutional and spastic entropion, since they can be performed quickly and yield immediate relief. This procedure simultaneously addresses the problems of retractor disinsertion/attenuation and overriding of the preseptal orbicularis. The sutures are placed deep in the fornix, aiming at the inferior orbital rim to ensure engagement of the disinserted retractors. The passage of the sutures induces a vector force that rotates the lid margin outward, and the resultant subcutaneous inflammatory cicatrix prevents the preseptal orbicularis from overriding the pretarsal orbicularis.

When used alone for entropion repair, fornix sutures have a recurrence rate of 9 to 33%.[23,24] The authors' preferred technique for correcting spastic entropion is to use fornix sutures in conjunction with a lateral tarsal strip. The recurrence rate for a combined procedure is 1.6%.[24] Furthermore, the authors have not encountered any postoperative ectropion with this combined approach.

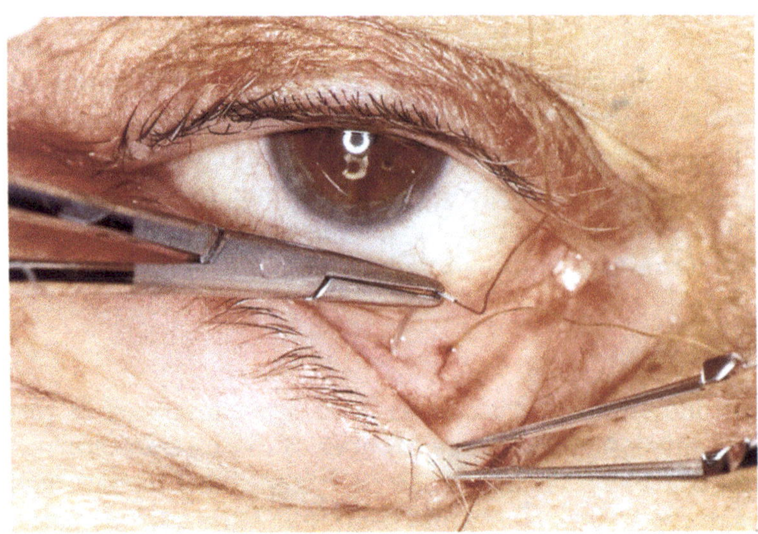

FIGURE 11.2. Placement of full-thickness eyelid sutures for entropion repair.

A drop of topical tetracaine is applied to the eye and a cotton pledget moistened with 4% lidocaine is placed in the inferior fornix for several minutes. This maneuver provides sufficient topical anesthesia, and discomfort of the needle stick through the conjunctiva is minimal. Lidocaine with epinephrine (1:100,000) is injected subconjunctivally by means of a 30-gauge needle.

The lower eyelid is pulled away from the globe with forceps. One needle of a double-armed 5-0 chromic suture is passed in a perpendicular fashion through the eyelid, beginning deep within the inferior fornix. The needle is aimed toward the orbital rim to ensure engagement of the retractors (Fig. 11.2).

The surgeon "tents" the skin about 1.5 cm from the lid margin and advances the needle superiorly under the skin. The needle penetrates the skin 3 to 4 mm below the lash line. The other arm of the suture is passed in an identical manner, parallel to the first arm, and exits the skin at the same horizontal level, within 5 to 6 mm. Two or three additional double-armed sutures are evenly placed in a similar fashion across the eyelid. When the arms of the sutures are tied over bolsters, they will evert the eyelid margin. By tightening the sutures more, the surgeon can cause greater eversion. A slight overcorrection is desirable. An inflammatory cicatrix will form and retain the eyelid in proper position (Fig. 11.3).

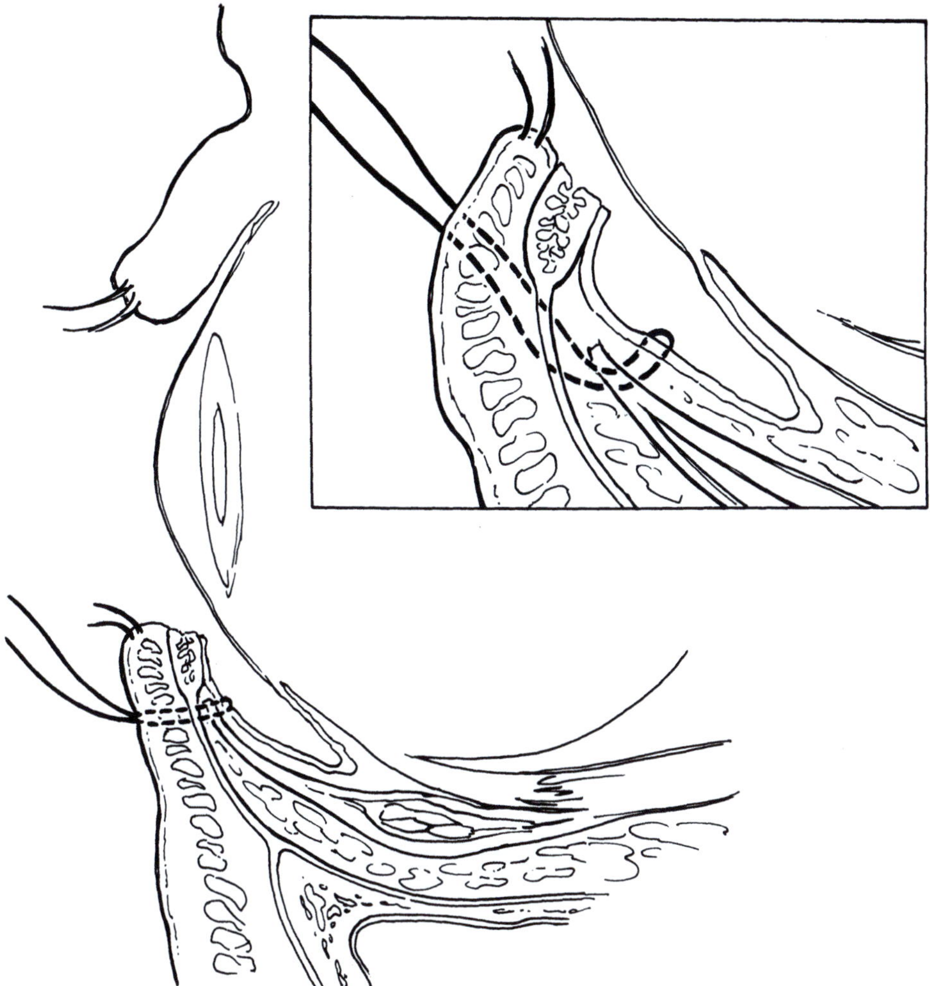

FIGURE 11.3. Sagittal view of suture passage through the lower eyelid: a slight overcorrection is desirable. (Reproduced with permission from Classification and treatment of eyelid malposition. In: Nesi FA, Gladstone JG, Brazzo BG, et al. eds. *Ophthalmic and Facial Plastic Surgery: A Compendium of Aesthetic and Reconstructive Techniques.* Thorofare, NJ: Slack Incorporated, 2000:88.)

Direct Repair of Lower Eyelid Retractors: Transcutaneous Approach

Direct repair of entropion with reinsertion of the lower eyelid retractors to the inferior tarsal border is commonly performed through a subciliary incision. This procedure is analogous to the aponeurotic ptosis repair of the upper eyelid, in which the disinserted aponeurosis is advanced onto the tarsal plate. This approach offers the opportunity to inspect the lower eyelid anatomy and provides access for removal of preaponeurotic fat and redundant skin. When performed alone, recurrence rates ranged from 0 to 5%.[25,26] Wesley and Collins reported no recurrences when a lateral tarsal strip was performed to address horizontal eyelid laxity.[12] Direct repair carries the disadvantage of being time-consuming and technically more difficult, and possibly causing secondary ectropion.[25] Boboridis et al. noted a 11% overcorrection when direct retractors reattachment was performed without simultaneous horizontal lid shortening.[25]

Dresner and Karesh[27] described the technique of transconjunctival approach to advance or fortify the lower eyelid retractors. Lateral canthal resuspension, transconjunctival blepharoplasty, and the position of the orbicularis muscle can all be addressed by this method. Dresner and Karesh reported no postoperative recurrences, overcorrections, or lower eyelid retraction with 9 to 18 months of follow-up.

A subciliary incision extending from just temporal to the lacrimal punctum to the lateral canthus is outlined with a marking pen. Topical tetracaine is applied. A subcutaneous injection of 2% lidocaine with epinephrine (1:100,000) is performed.

A 4-0 silk traction suture is placed centrally in a horizontal lamellar fashion through the tarsal plate of the lower eyelid margin. This suture is anchored to the surgical drape superiorly to place the posterior lamella on stretch, while permitting mobilization of the anterior lamella.

Subciliary incision is made with a blade, and a skin–muscle flap is developed. The surgeon should enter the avascular postorbicular fascial plane. Relaxing incisions are made medially and laterally with Westcott scissors. Meticulous hemostasis throughout the procedure by means of bipolar cautery optimizes visualization of the anatomic landmarks.

Gentle pressure is applied to the globe to prolapse the preaponeurotic fat pads forward. As in upper lid surgery, the orbital fat pads are the key anatomical landmarks to identify, since the retractors are situated beneath (superior to) the fat pads. The orbital septum is el-

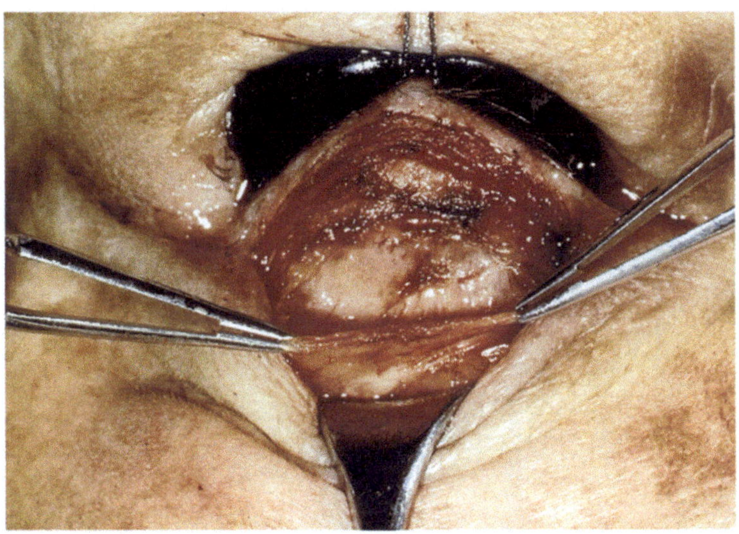

FIGURE 11.4. Reattachment of eyelid retractors. Forceps are holding the disinserted edge of the retractors. Anatomically, the capsulopalpebral fascia is verified by its location beneath the preaponeurotic fat.

evated with forceps and incised with blunt Westcott scissors. The orbital fat pads are gently dissected off the white glistening anterior surface of the retractors. The structure is then inspected for dehiscence or disinsertion. Frequently, the disinserted edge is apparent. Anatomically, the capsulopalpebral fascia is verified by its location beneath the preaponeurotic fat (Fig. 11.4). Physiologically, this structure can be further verified by instructing the patient to look downward while engaging the edge with forceps. The retractors should generate a force with downward movement.

The disinserted edge of the retractors is then reattached onto the inferior margin of the tarsus by means of a 5-0 Vicryl suture

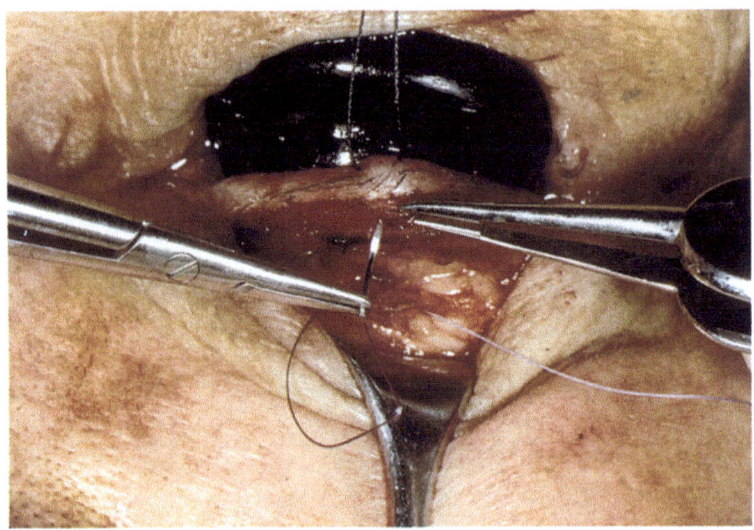

FIGURE 11.5. The disinserted edge of the retractors is reattached to the inferior margin of the tarsus by means of 5-0 Vicryl sutures.

(Fig. 11.5). The surgeon should avoid suturing the retractors to the anterior surface of the tarsal plate because this may induce lid margin eversion. With proper suture placement, the eyelid demonstrates smooth excursion with downgaze.

Several interrupted sutures are placed in an identical fashion to secure the retractors to the tarsal plate. Excess orbital fat can be clamped with a hemostat and excised. Frequently, concomitant horizontal eyelid laxity is present, requiring a lateral tarsal strip procedure (see Chapter 10).

Occasionally, following an eyelid-shortening procedure, the tarsal plate will not be long enough to reach the periosteum of the lateral orbital rim. Attempting to tighten the eyelid in this scenario may cause the lid to glide under the equator of the globe. Alternatively, the lid margin may turn inward, further exacerbating eye irritation. In this situation, a periosteal flap measuring 4×6 mm^2 is fashioned on the outer surface of the lateral orbital rim. The flap is reflected nasally to unite with the temporal end of the tarsal plate. A 5-0 Mersilene mattress suture is used to secure these structures.

A small amount of excess skin can be removed from the inferior edge of the incision. The lower lid incision is closed with a running 6-0 suture. The traction suture is removed.

Entropion

Marginal Rotation, with Full-Thickness Blepharotomy

Rotation of the eyelid margin can be utilized for involutional and mild to moderate cases of cicatricial entropion. A full-thickness horizontal incision disinserts all attachments of the lower eyelid at the level of the inferior border of the tarsal plate. The transverse full-thickness defect is repaired by transferring the eversion effect of the lower eyelid retractors to the anterior lamella of the lid margin bridge flap. This technique promotes a well-defined scar tissue barrier to shorten the retractors, evert the tarsal plate, and inhibit upward overriding of the preseptal orbicularis muscle. A recurrence rate of 11 to 17%, and overcorrection of 31% has been documented during the treatment of involutional entropion.[25,28] Millman et al. reported a recurrence rate of 7% and overcorrection of 5% in patients treated for cicatricial entropion.[29]

A modification of this procedure is used in the upper lid for mild to moderate cicatricial entropion.[30] A full-thickness horizontal upper eyelid incision is made 4 mm above the lid margin. The posterior lamella is united with the anterior lamella of the bridge flap to effect eversion of the lid margin.

A horizontal incision is outlined with a marking pen on the upper lid, 4 to 5 mm from the margin. The incision marking should begin 1 to 2 mm temporal to the punctum, extending to the lateral canthal angle. If only a small area of the lid requires repair, the incision may be made smaller to correspond to the entropion. Topical tetracaine is applied and a cotton pledget moistened with 4% lidocaine is placed in the fornix prior to subconjunctival infiltration with 2% lidocaine with epinephrine (1:100,000). A small amount of anesthetic is also injected subcutaneously across the entire eyelid.

A 4-0 silk traction suture is placed through the tarsal plate of the lid margin near the medial and temporal limbus. This suture is retracted inferiorly and a lid plate is placed in the superior fornix to protect the globe. Alternatively, a large chalazion clamp can be used for eyelid fixation. However, shallow fornix or symblepharon may preclude its use.

A transverse skin incision is made through the tarsal plate over the preplaced marking with a #15 Bard–Parker blade. The blade should be placed perpendicular to the plane of the lid and parallel to the lid margin. The incision extends through the pretarsal orbicularis until the epitarsal surface is visualized. Good hemostasis helps the surgeon to identify this landmark.

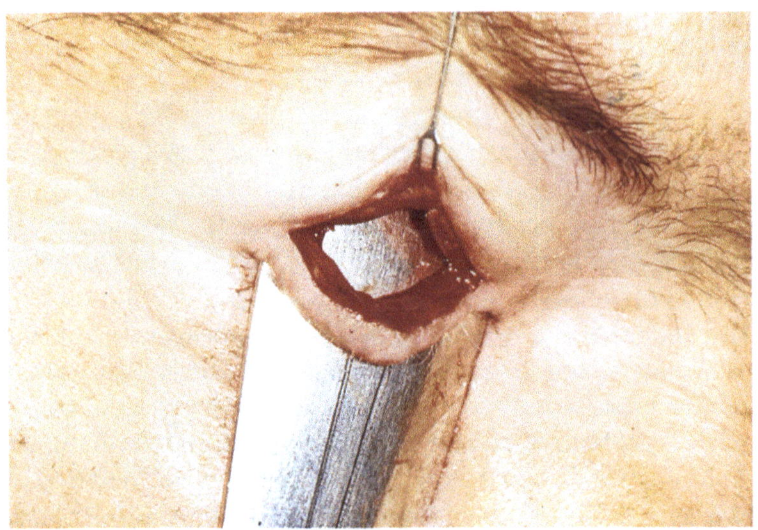

FIGURE 11.6. Full-thickness eyelid incision through the tarsal plate is made with the scalpel blade. The incision is extended laterally to the temporal end of the tarsal plate with Stevens scissors, and medially to just lateral to the lacrimal punctum.

A full-thickness incision through the tarsal plate is made with the blade (Fig. 11.6). The incision is extended in both directions with Stevens scissors. The surgeon should not extend the incision beyond the tarsal plate proper, to avoid severing the palpebral arterial supply.

Both arms of a double-armed 5-0 Vicryl suture are passed in a lamellar fashion through the superior tarsal stump. Two or three additional double-armed sutures are placed 3 to 4 mm apart (Fig. 11.7). Each pair may be tagged with clamps to avoid confusion. The needle arms are passed through the bridge flap in a plane just anterior to the tarsus and posterior to the pretarsal orbicularis muscle. The sutures then exit through the orbicularis and skin 2 mm above the lash line.

All three sets of suture should be evenly spaced along the full-thickness incision prior to closure of the skin edges (Fig. 11.8). The skin incision is closed with a 6-0 running nylon or gut suture.

Each double-armed suture is tied over a small cotton bolster, which serves as a fulcrum for everting the lid margin. Slight overcorrection is desired. The everting sutures and cotton bolsters are removed in 2 weeks. An antibiotic ointment is applied three times a day during this period.

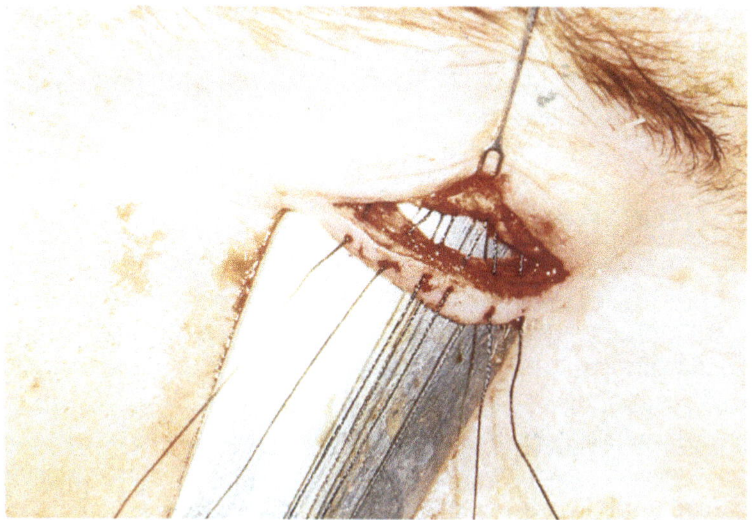

FIGURE 11.7. Double-armed 5-0 Vicryl sutures are passed in a lamellar fashion through the superior tarsal stump. The needle arms are passed through the inferior bridge flap in a plane just anterior to the tarsus and posterior to the pretarsal orbicularis muscle. The sutures then exit through the orbicularis and skin, 2 mm above the lash line.

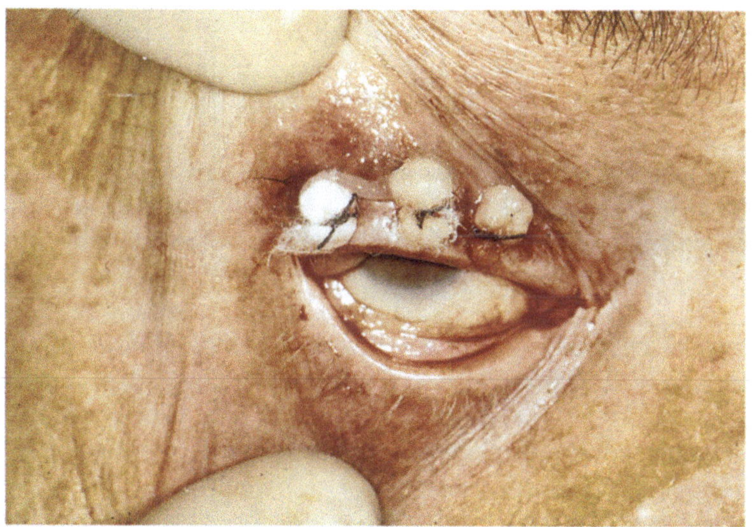

FIGURE 11.8. All three sets of sutures are evenly spaced along the full-thickness incision prior to closure of the skin edges. The skin incision is closed with a 6-0 running nylon or gut suture.

This procedure may also be used in the lower lid for repair of mild to moderate cicatricial entropion. The blepharotomy is made near the inferior tarsal border, about 4 mm from the margin. The everting sutures are placed in a similar fashion.

COMPLICATIONS

Fornix suture placement alone is associated with a recurrence rate of 9 to 33%.[23,24] This high rate of recurrence is principally due to a failure to recognize concomitant horizontal laxity. A simultaneous horizontal tightening procedure can significantly decrease this rate and minimize eyelid retraction. Suture advancement of the lower eyelid retractors in conjunction with a lateral tarsal strip procedure is an efficient, physiological, and effective approach in achieving long-lasting correction for involutional entropion, since all three elements of pathology are addressed. The lateral tarsal strip procedure corrects horizontal laxity and maintains the almond-shaped canthal angle, while avoiding phimosis and lid notching. This combination approach is the authors' preferred method of treatment for involutional entropion.

A mild overcorrection intraoperatively is preferred when full-thickness sutures or marginal rotation is used. However, overcorrection is the most commonly cited complication of the marginal rotation procedure. Fortunately, the amount and location of lid eversion can be modified at the time of surgery. If the sutures are placed through the anterior lamella too close to the lid margin, the everting forces are maximized and ectropion and punctal eversion may occur. If the sutures are placed too far from the lid margin, minimal rotation will result.[31] Postoperatively, overcorrection can be addressed by removing one or more sutures at the 1-week visit and massaging the lid.

Ectropion may also occur after direct reattachment of the lower lid retractors if the retractors are sutured to the anterior tarsal surface, rather than to the inferior border of the tarsus. A horizontal tightening procedure performed at the same time should minimize the incidence of lid malposition.

Eyelid retraction and scleral show are possible if excessive shortening or advancement of the retractors occurs. Close monitoring of the relative position of the lid to the globe during the procedure will minimize this complication. Excessive removal of lower eyelid skin may also exaggerate this effect and should be avoided.

Eyelid margin necrosis may occur following a marginal rotation procedure if the marginal vascular arcade is severed at both ends. The full-thickness eyelid incision should be placed at or below the inferior border of the lower tarsus, and in the upper lid at least 4 to 5 mm from the margin to avoid vascular compromise. Fistula formation may occur in the lid-splitting procedure and can be corrected by excision.[32] A single case of central corneal dellen formation was reported as a complication of an upper eyelid tarsotomy for cicatricial entropion. A buckled tarsal plate, formed by premature separation of the tarsoconjunctival flap, produced suboptimal lid–globe apposition during lid closure. The pathogenesis of central dellen was thought to be due to an abnormal tear meniscus under the buckled central eyelid, inducing focal corneal dehydration. Proper lid–globe apposition should be assessed at the completion of a marginal rotation procedure to avoid this complication.[33]

REFERENCES

1. Fox SA. The etiology of senile entropion. *Am J Ophthalmol* 1959;48:607–611.

2. Jones LT. The anatomy of the lower eyelid and its relation to the cause and care of entropion. *Am J Ophthalmol* 1960;42:29–36.

3. Jones LT, Reeh MJ, Tsujimura JK. Senile entropion. *Am J Ophthalmol* 1963;55:463–469.

4. Levine MR. Involutional entropion. *Ophthalmic Pract* 1987;5:118–139.

5. Benger RS, Musch DC. A comparative study of eyelid parameters in involutional entropion. *Ophthalmic Plast Reconstr Surg* 1989;5:281–287.

6. Dalgleish R, Smith JLS. Mechanics and histology of senile entropion. *Br J Ophthalmol* 1966;50:79–91.

7. Schaeffer A. Involutional entropion. In: Smith BC, Della Rocca RC, Nesi FA, Lisman RD, eds. *Ophthalmic Plastic and Reconstructive Surgery*. Vol 1. St Louis: Mosby-Year Book; 1987:550.

8. Bick MW. Surgical management of orbital tarsal disparity. *Arch Ophthalmol* 1966;75:386–389.

9. Martin RT, Nunery WR, Tannebaum M. Entropion, trichiasis, and distichiasis. In: McCord CD, Tanenbaum M, Nunery WR, eds. *Oculoplastic Surgery*. 3d. ed. New York: Raven Press; 1995:221–230.

10. Rainin EA. Senile entropion. *Arch Ophthalmol* 1979;97:928–930.

11. Jackson ST. Surgery for involutional entropion. *Ophthalmic Surg* 1983;14:322–326.

12. Wesley RE, Collins JW. Combined procedure for senile entropion. *Ophthalmic Surg* 1983;14:401–405.

13. Schaefer AJ. Variation in the pathophysiology of involutional entropion and its treatment. *Ophthalmic Surg* 1983;14:653–655.

14. Jones L, Reed MJ, Wobig JL. Senile entropion: a new concept for correction. *Am J Ophthalmol* 1972;74:327–329.

15. Collin JRO, Rathbun JE. Involutional entropion. *Arch Ophthalmol* 1978;96:1058–1064.

16. Dryden RM, Leibsohn J, Wobig JL. Senile entropion: pathogenesis and treatment. *Arch Ophthalmol* 1978;96:1883–1885.

17. Hargiss JL. Inferior aponeurosis vs orbital septum tucking for senile entropion. *Arch Ophthalmol* 1973;89:210–213.

18. Hawes MJ, Dortzbach RK. The microscopic anatomy of the lower eyelid retractors. *Arch Ophthalmol* 1982;100:1313–1318.

19. Dortzbach RK, McGetrick JJ. Involutional entropion of the lower eyelid. *Adv Ophthalmic Plast Reconstr Surg* 1983;2:257–267.

20. Feldstein M. Suture correction of senile entropion by inferior lid retractor tuck. *Adv Ophthalmic Plast Reconstr Surg* 1983;2:269–274.

21. Carter SR, Chang J, Aguilar GL, Rathbun JE, Seiff SR. Involutional entropion and ectropion of the Asian lower eyelid. *Ophthalmic Plast Reconstr Surg* 2000;16:45–49.

22. Markovits AS. Variations on the theme of involutional entropion and Quickert repair. *Ann Ophthalmol* 1980;12:1028–1040.

23. Iliff NT. An easy approach to entropion surgery. *Ann Ophthalmol* 1976;8:1343–1346.

24. Rougraff PM, Tse DT, Johnson TE, Feuer W. Involutional entropion repair with fornix sutures and lateral tarsal strip procedure. *Ophthalmic Plast Reconstr Surgery*. 2001:17(4):281–287.

25. Boboridis K, Bunce C, Rose GE. A comparative study of two procedures for repair of involutional lower lid entropion. *Ophthalmology* 2000;7(5):959–961.

26. Caldato R, Lauande-Pimentel R, Sabrosa NA, Fonseca RA, Paiva RS, Alves MR, Jose NK. Role of reinsertion of the lower eyelid retractor on involutional entropion. *Br J Ophthalmol* 2000;84(6):606–608.

27. Dresner SC, Karesh JW. Transconjunctival entropion repair. *Arch Ophthalmol* 1993;111:1144–1148.

28. Lance SE, Wilkins RB. Involutional entropion: a retrospective analysis of the Wies procedure alone or combined with a horizontal shortening procedure. *Ophthalmic Plast Reconstr Surg* 1991;7(4):273–277.

29. Millman AL, Katzen LB, Putterman AM. Cicatricial entropion: an analysis of its treatment with transverse blepharotomy and marginal rotation. *Ophthalmic Plast Reconstr Surg* 1989;20(8):575–579.

30. Ballen PH. A simple procedure for the relief of trichiasis and entropion of the upper lid. *Arch Ophthalmol* 1964;72:239–240.

31. Baylis HI, Cies WA, Kamin DF. Overcorrections of the Wies procedure. *Ann Ophthalmol* 1977;9(6):744–748.

32. Custer PL. Eyelid fistula following Wies entropion repair. *Ophthalmic Surg* 1988;19(6):417–418.

33. Kwok SK, Tse DT. Central corneal dellen: a complication of upper eyelid tarsotomy. *Ophthalmic Plast Reconstr Surg* 2000;16(3)237–240.

BIBLIOGRAPHY

Quickert MH, Rathbun E. Suture repair of entropion. *Arch Ophthalmol* 1971;85: 304–305.

Tse DT. In: Wright KW, ed. *Color Atlas of Ophthalmic Surgery: Oculoplastic Surgery.* Philadelphia: Lippincott; 1992.

Wies FA. Spastic entropion. *Trans Am Acad Ophthalmol Otolaryngol* 1955;59:503.

12

EYELID RETRACTION

• Richard A. Stangler

Eyelid retraction results from a multitude of different etiologies including thyroid-related, inflammatory, mechanical, and traumatic causes. Once a diagnosis of functionally or cosmetically significant retraction has been made, treatment can be planned. The primary focus of the lid retraction evaluation is to determine the lamellar level of pathology.

EVALUATION

The eyelid is separated anatomically into the anterior, middle, and posterior lamellae. The anterior lamella is typically defined as the skin and orbicularis muscle. The middle lamella includes the levator aponeurosis, Muller's muscle, and orbital septum in the upper lid, and the eyelid retractors and orbital septum in the lower eyelid. The posterior lamella consists of the tarsus and conjunctiva. Pathology in one or more or these layers may be the source of lid retraction. Usually, the main goal of the evaluation is to differentiate anterior lamellar retraction, which may occur in burn or post–facial surgery patients,[1] from retraction secondary to more posterior pathology, which is most common in thyroid-related cases.

The patient's history is paramount in determining the cause of lid retraction and will likely point the physician to the source of the problem. The exam should then be confirmatory.

A full ophthalmic exam includes measurements of lagophthalmos, MRD1 and MRD2 (distances from the corneal light reflex to the upper lid and lower lid margins, respectively), and SS1 and SS2 (scleral show between the corneal limbus and superior and inferior lid margins, respectively). The author prefers three additional tests to confirm the level of pathology and determine the mode of treatment.

The first is the "vertical eyelid elevation test," which is done with eyes closed for upper lid retraction and eyes open for lower lid retraction. It involves placing the finger on the affected lid and pushing down on the upper lid or up on the lower lid. A deficiency in the anterior lamella will be perceived as skin tautness with vertical skin tension lines (Fig. 12.1A). If, instead, the skin moves in the intended direction by sliding over the posterior levels while the lid remains tethered in position, the pathology is posterior to the skin and orbicularis (Fig. 12.1B).

Second, an anterior lamellar shortage can further be verified by having the patient open his or her mouth. With normal skin laxity, there should be no increase in retraction; with an anterior lamellar shortage, the retraction tends to worsen. Finally, for cases of mild lower lid retraction, the "sweep" test is performed. The examiner places a finger just lateral of the central point on the lower lid and sweeps up and out. If the eyelid returns to its natural position, the retraction can likely be repaired with a tarsal strip and canthoplasty. Otherwise, a more aggressive surgical approach is required.

This chapter will concentrate on the repair of middle ($\pm$posterior) lamellar retraction that may be seen in patients with thyroid disease or with prominent involutional "retraction" of the lower lids accompanied by symptoms of irritation or tearing.

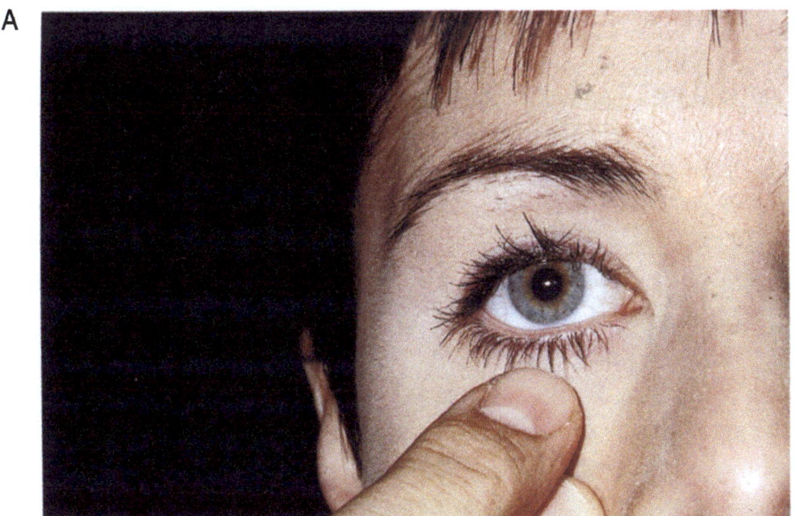

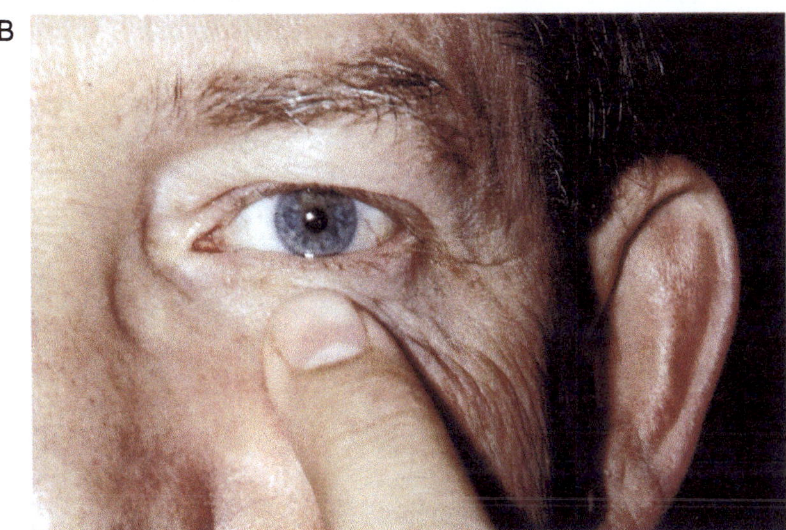

FIGURE 12.1. The vertical eyelid elevation test. (A) A patient 15 years after transcutaneous blepharoplasty, with tearing and mild lagophthalmos. (B) The skin easily moves in the intended direction by sliding over the posterior levels while the tarsus remains tethered in position, indicating that the pathology is posterior to the skin and orbicularis. A deficiency in the anterior lamella would be perceived as skin tautness, with vertical skin tension lines.

TECHNIQUES

Upper Eyelid Retraction, Anterior (External) Approach

This section describes the author's preferred anterior approach for thyroid-related upper eyelid retraction. It is important for the patient's ocular exam to have shown extended stability, ideally 6 months or longer, to avoid recurrent problems after repair. Orbital decompression, if deemed necessary, is typically performed as a primary procedure in the thyroid patient. Anticipated eye muscle surgery should be done prior to eyelid retraction repair because the recession of the vertical rectus muscles increases eyelid retraction of the adjacent involved lids.[2] The author typically prefers the anterior approach when there is an anticipated concomitant excision of anterior lamellar tissue, or orbital or sub-brow fat because it allows easy access.

In performing anterior upper lid retraction repair, a felt-tipped pen is used to mark the eyelid crease and the area of redundant anterior lamellar tissue that will be excised with blepharoplasty. It is important to place these markings before injection, since the anesthetic will distort the lid landmarks. An anesthetic composed of an equal volume of 2% lidocaine with epinephrine and 0.75% bupivicaine is injected subcutaneously to the involved areas. A small amount of the local anesthetic is given centrally along the lid margin where a traction suture will be placed. The tissue is lightly massaged with 4 × 4 sponge to spread the anesthetic fluid through tissue planes.

A 4-0 silk traction suture is passed through the lid margin centrally. Next a #15 Bard–Parker blade is used to incise the skin and orbicularis muscle. The redundant anterior lamellar tissue is removed, exposing the septum.

At this point, the surgeon's orientation will be aided greatly by locating the superior tarsal plate. This is done by first dissecting the skin and orbicularis muscle from the middle lamella between the lid margin and crease. Care must be taken not to carry this dissection within 2 to 3 mm of the margin to avoid trauma to the lash follicles. The superior tarsus is exposed by excising pretarsal orbicularis muscle. During this maneuver, the levator aponeurosis over the anterior tarsus, and the epitarsal tissue, are also excised.

If orbital fat removal is planned, the septum is tented and incised horizontally. The preaponeurotic fat is exposed, along with the underlying levator muscle and aponeurosis. Fat pads are removed as desired. The levator muscle is then released from the superior border of the tarsus with scissors or cautery. The patient's lid height may be checked at this point; however, in all but minimal retraction cases, Muller's muscle will need to be recessed as well.

The author waits until this point in the surgery to evert the lid over a Desmarres retractor and inject the local anesthetic solution subconjunctivally. Hydraulic dissection between the conjunctiva and Muller's muscle greatly facilitates the following dissection and also provides an additional fluid "buffer" over the anterior surface of the eye. Mild traction is placed inferiorly on the 4-0 silk suture.

Muller's muscle is released from the superior border of the tarsus. While holding Muller's muscle with a fine forceps and pulling slightly upward and toward the patient's head, the author prefers to release the muscle with a disposable hot cautery. Cautery is used rather than scissors because the Muller's muscle is quite vascular and otherwise tends to bleed copiously.

Dissection should be carried to the lateral part of the tarsus to avoid lateral canthal "flaring" or undercorrection. Lacrimal gland tissue may be encountered during the performance of this dissection; extensive dissection through lacrimal tissue should be avoided, even if retraction persists. The author generally only releases the temporal two-thirds of Muller's muscle. Medial overcorrection is a common complication of retraction repair.

The patient should be placed in the sitting position to judge lid height. A significant recession of approximately 8 mm is performed for the typical retraction case, generally yielding 2 to 3 mm of correction. The goal is an overcorrection of 1 to 2 mm from desired lid height, allowing for postoperative raising of the lid. Portions of Muller's muscle may be reattached to the superior tarsus if overcorrection occurs. The attachment is placed centrally if the lid contour has flattened.

A lateral tarsorrhaphy is frequently useful as an adjunctive procedure for significant retraction cases to diminish the lateral undercorrection or "flaring." In addition, moving the canthus medially often affords a significant reduction in the perceived exophthalmos from the lateral view.

Once the desired height has been obtained, the skin is closed with 6-0 mild chromic suture. The traction suture is secured to the cheek and left in place for 24 to 48 hours for unilateral procedures. Postoperatively, cold packs are recommended for 15 minutes every hour for several hours to help reduce swelling.

Upper Eyelid Retraction, Posterior (Internal) Approach

The posterior conjunctival approach is the author's preferred approach for upper eyelid retraction, particularly if there is no associated skin, orbital fat, or sub-brow fat to remove. It also is preferred when combined with a minimal anterior lamellar excision.

Local anesthetic comprising an equal volume of 2% lidocaine with epinephrine and 0.75% bupivicaine is injected into the retracted lid both subcutaneously and subconjunctivally. Total anesthetic fluid volume is minimized to avoid significantly altering the eyelid position or levator function. The tissue is then massaged lightly with a 4 × 4 sponge for a few minutes to spread the infiltrate.

A 4-0 silk traction suture is placed centrally in the lid margin. The lid is everted over a Desmarres retractor. With the temporal conjunctiva tented with a small-toothed forceps, a snip incision is made with Westcott scissors over the superior tarsal border. The conjunctiva is carefully undermined with scissors along the entire superior tarsal border, to separate conjunctiva from Muller's muscle (Fig. 12.2). With assistant and surgeon each grasping one side of the conjunctiva, and the tissue placed on mild tension, the intervening conjunctiva is cleared of remaining Muller's muscle attachments to the superior fornix.

This dissection is aided by spreading the scissors carefully against the conjunctiva while observing the tips of the scissors through the transparent conjunctiva. Care must be taken to avoid buttonholes, although these typically are not repaired if they occur. It is important to release Muller's muscle extensively because any remaining slip attachments tend to impair the final result.

The next step is to separate Muller's muscle from the tarsus and the levator muscle. As with the external retraction repair, Muller's muscle release is performed over the temporal two-thirds of the lid only, to prevent medial overcorrection. Therefore, Muller's muscle is grasped with forceps at the temporal end near the initial supratarsal incision, and incised along the superior tarsal border with Westcott scissors. Moist cotton-tipped applicators are used to separate Muller's muscle from the loosely attached levator muscle and aponeurosis. Muller's muscle is dissected for approximately 10 mm above the superior tarsal border toward the superior fornix.

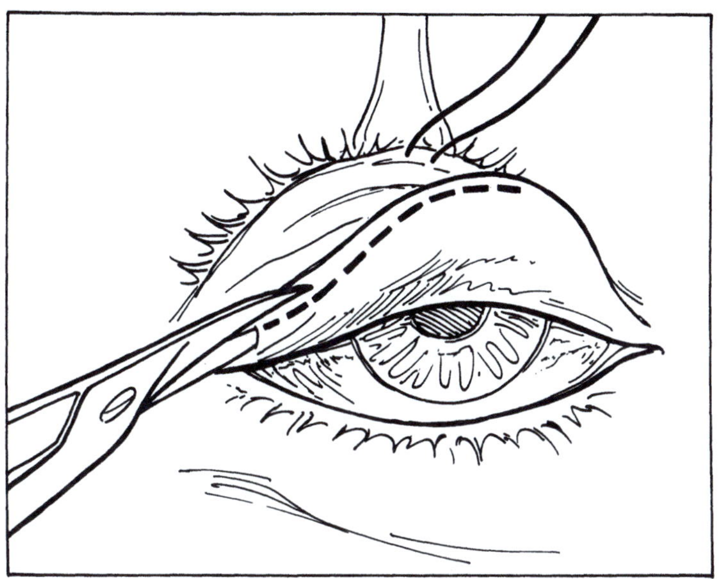

FIGURE 12.2. Incision of conjunctiva at superior tarsal border for the upper lid posterior retraction repair. (Reproduced with permission from Classification and treatment of eyelid malposition. In: Nesi FA, Gladstone GJ, Brazzo BG, et al, eds. *Ophthalmic and Facial Plastic Surgery: A Compendium of Reconstructive and Aesthetic Techniques.* Thorofare, NJ: Slack Incorporated; 2000:103.)

The patient is checked in the sitting position. A 1 to 2 mm overcorrection is preferred. Depending on the result, further release of Muller's muscle for another 2 to 4 mm can be performed. The lid height should be checked following each adjustment with the patient sitting.

Although the Muller's muscle could be left in place at the newly recessed level, the author finds that total excision of the muscle provides optimum results. This is accomplished by clamping the muscle with a small straight hemostat and incising the muscle with cautery while the muscle is placed on slight tension. These two steps help to ensure that the muscle does not bleed excessively.

If additional retraction release is required, the levator should be gradual lengthened. This is done in a titrated fashion by using two

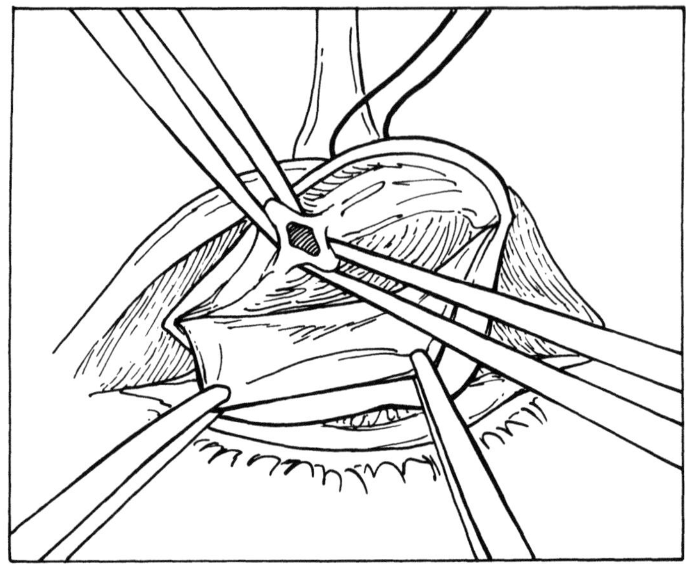

FIGURE 12.3. The levator aponeurosis is lengthened just superior to tarsus to adjust lid height and contour. (Reproduced with permission from Classification and treatment of eyelid malposition. In: Nesi FA, Gladstone GJ, Brazzo BG, et al, eds. *Ophthalmic and Facial Plastic Surgery: A Compendium of Reconstructive and Aesthetic Techniques.* Thorofare, NJ: Slack Incorporated; 2000:103.)

toothed forceps and separating aponeurosis tissue vertically, just superior to the tarsal border (Fig. 12.3). Obvious focal areas of retraction are addressed first but generally, in the author's hands, the entire temporal two-thirds of the lid requires at least one additional release.

The surgeon needs to develop a "feel" for this portion of the operation. If too much tissue is grasped, either vertically or horizontally, lengthening is difficult. The surgeon should be able to gently "shred" or separate the muscle fibers. Care must be taken to observe the aponeurosis after each lengthening maneuver, as the orbicularis and skin can be grasped and inadvertently shredded.

Eyelid Retraction

After a desired level for lid height has been reached, the conjunctiva can be closed with three buried 6-0 plain gut sutures. In unilateral procedures, the 4-0 silk traction suture is secured to the cheek for 24 to 48 hours. Ice is placed postoperatively for 15 minutes every hour for several hours.

Lower Eyelid Retraction

The repair of lower lid retraction depends on the extent and nature of the problem. For symptomatic patients with mild retraction, most will have marked laxity. It is important to differentiate this involutional subtype from those patients with a "tether" (scar) component.

The "sweep" test (ability of surgeon to place lid in proper position by gently elevating with a finger) determines whether a tarsal strip, combined with release of lower lid retractors, and possibly also a tarsorrhaphy, is adequate to correct the problem. If a more extensive remedy is needed, a spacer material can be used to help ensure an excellent result. The choice of spacers is varied, but the author prefers processed and screened cadaveric dermal allograft (AlloDerm, Life Cell Corp., The Woodlands, TX) for its texture and ease of use in moderate lower lid retraction cases.

For more severe cases, the surgeon should use a less pliable material. Autologous ear cartilage is usually the author's donor material of choice. Ease of harvest and cosmetically acceptable results make it a very useful tissue for repair. Although sometimes thought of as thick and difficult to manipulate, with proper preparation ear cartilege is an appropriate donor tissue for the majority of severe retraction cases. Many other types of spacer materials are successfully used for retraction repair by other surgeons including eye bank sclera, autologous nasal septal cartilage, hard palate mucosa, and molded porous polyethylene (Porex Surgical, College Park, GA).[2-4]

Before starting, it is imperative to have accurate measurements of the scleral show (SS) for each eyelid. Because the "natural" position of the lower eyelid is at or about the lower limbus, the SS2 generally indicates the significance of the retraction. Of course, the de-

---

sired outcome should be modified to suit the individual situation as determined, for instance, by old photographs or the level of difference in unilateral cases.

Preoperatively, the author finds it useful to measure the level of retraction in dim rather than bright light to prevent the inadvertent "squinting" by the patient, which lessens the level of scleral show (Fig. 12.4A). Proper lighting often elicits an additional millimeter or more of latent retraction. Failure to account for this discrepancy can lead to surgical undercorrection.

A local injection of equal volumes of 2% lidocaine with epinephrine and 0.75% bupivicaine is given to the lateral canthus area just inside the lateral orbital rim, subconjunctivally along the length of the lower lid, and to the central eyelid just inferior to the lashes. If ear cartilage is to be used, subcutaneous injections are also given to the proposed donor site.

A 4-0 silk traction suture is placed in the central lower lid along the margin. Lateral canthotomy and inferior cantholysis are performed with Westcott scissors. The lid is everted over a Desmarres retractor. Westcott scissors are used to sever the conjunctiva and lower lid retractors at the inferior tarsal border. A dissection is carried out between the retractor and orbicularis muscles.

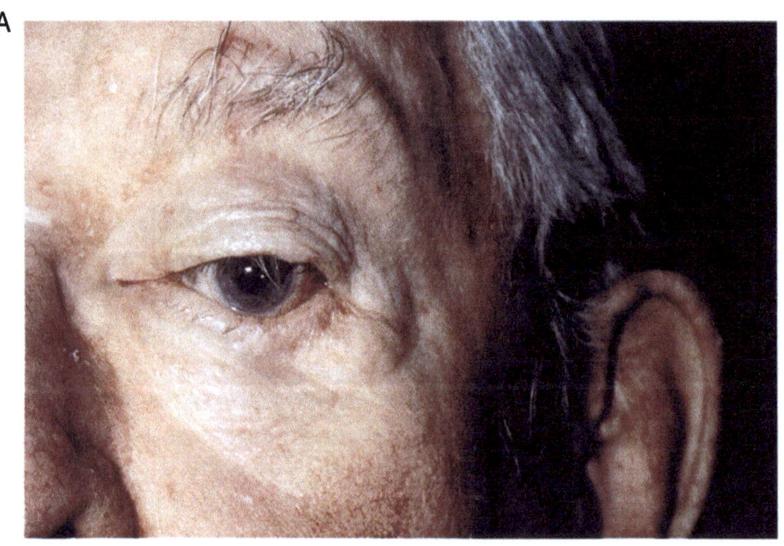

FIGURE 12.4. Typical involutional "retraction." (A) Preoperative left lower eyelid retraction.

Eyelid Retraction

Because the success of the procedure may be influenced significantly by bleeding between the graft and orbicularis muscle, meticulous hemostasis is important. The author prefers to use handheld cautery for dissection and recession of the retractors and conjunctiva.

The type of graft choice dictates the next few steps of the procedure (also see Chapter 9 for graft placement technique). For cases of severe retraction, ear cartilage is harvested by first marking with a felt-tipped pen along the posterior helix. A skin incision is then made with a #15 Bard–Parker blade. Westcott scissors are used to dissect between the skin and cartilage to expose a large, flat area of cartilage (Fig. 12.4B). The donor cartilage is marked to the desired width and 25 mm in length with a felt-tipped pen. The author finds that the graft yields best results when the width is approximately 1.5 times the desired height improvement. The cartilage graft is then incised around its borders with a #15 blade and harvested with Westcott scissors. The skin is closed with a running 6-0 mild chromic suture.

The ear cartilage is then prepared meticulously for implantation (Fig. 12.4C). First the graft is debrided of the epicartilagenous tissues. In the process, pressure is placed downward with the Westcott scissors on the graft to make both sides as thin as possible. Next, the graft is "scored" on one side by making both vertical and horizontal

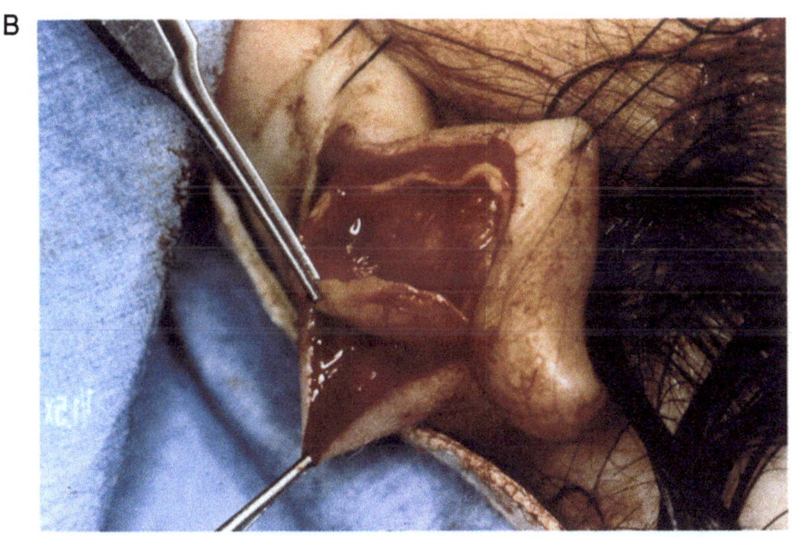

FIGURE 12.4. (B) Ear cartilage is harvested.

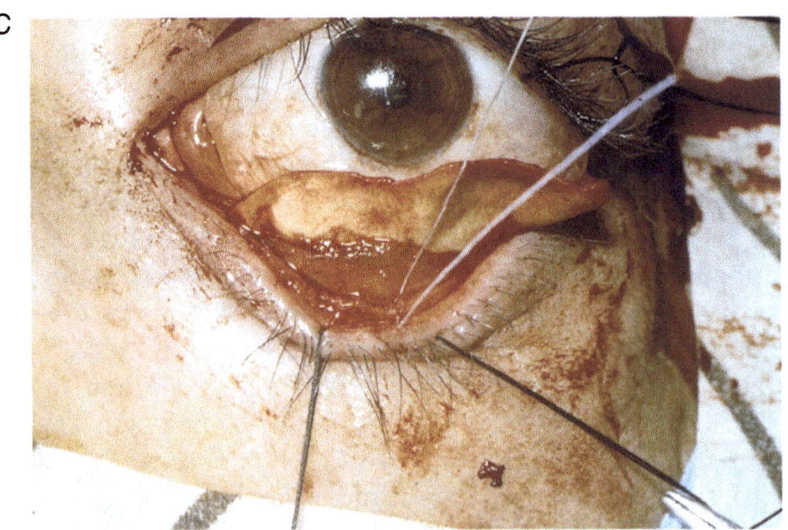

FIGURE 12.4. (C) Ear cartilage graft is measured to lower eyelid deficit, prepared, and secured to the recipient bed with simple interrupted 6-0 plain gut sutures.

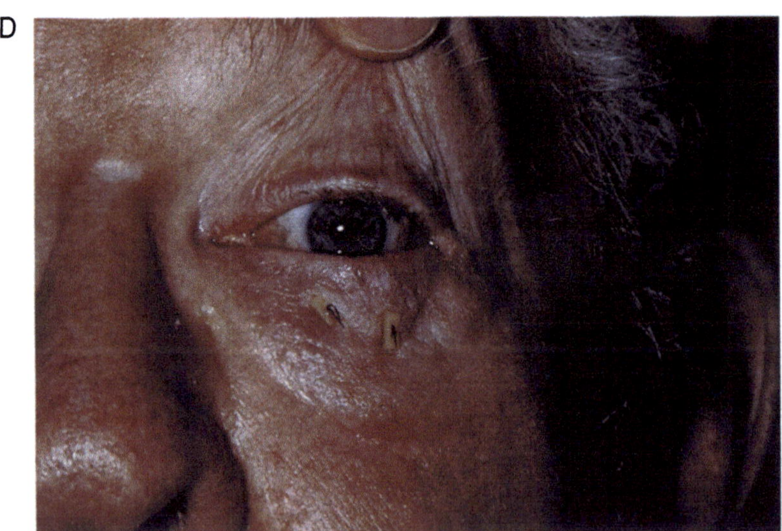

FIGURE 12.4. (D) Five days postoperative; the 6-0 silk sutures and rubber band bolsters are removed at 10 to 12 days.

partial-thickness striations with the #15 blade. This step is done assiduously, with striations every half millimeter, and will produce a pliable graft with adequate vertical strength.

After the graft has been sutured to its recipient site with 6-0 gut sutures, the author employs a second means of fixation. Two double-armed silk sutures are placed from posterior to anterior through the graft and the lid. These sutures are then passed through and tied over a rubber band bolster (Fig. 12.4D).

A lateral tarsal strip is developed (see Chapter 10). The surgeon should remember to remove the conjunctiva from the posterior surface with a blade, to avoid the formation of epithelial inclusion cysts. The tarsal strip is secured to the periosteum of the lateral orbital rim using a 5-0 Prolene mattress suture.

When securing the tarsal strip to the periosteum, it is important to place the suture slightly (1–2 mm) within the orbital rim to mimic the normal canthal attachment to the lateral tubercle. Failure to do this can result in eyelid malposition, which "lifts" the lid away from the globe as it passes laterally to the canthus. It is also important to place the suture slightly higher (1–1.5 mm) than the expected result to allow for postoperative regression (Fig. 12.5).

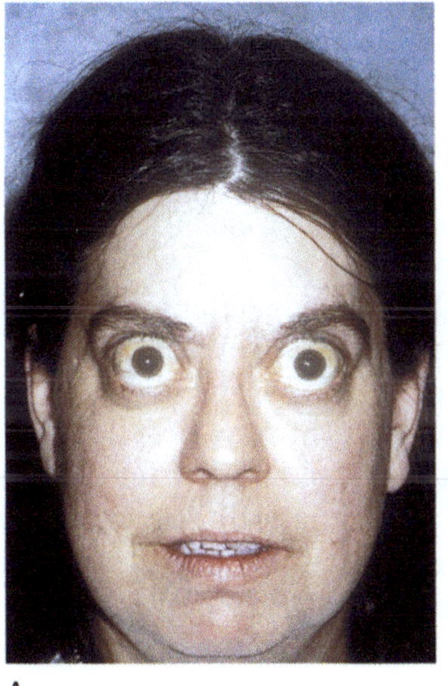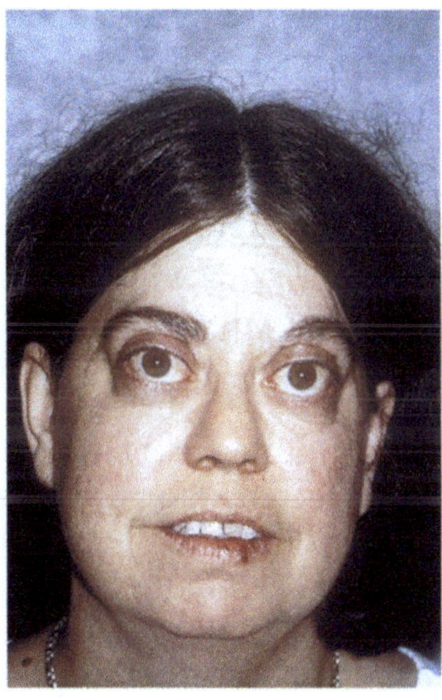

A   B

FIGURE 12.5. (A) Patient with severe eyelid retraction, secondary to thyroid-related ophthalmopathy. (B) Patient following upper lid internal repair and lower lid cartilage grafts.

The lateral canthal angle and skin are re-formed by using 6-0 mild chromic suture. The author places an antibiotic–steroid ointment on the eyes to help with postoperative comfort and then secures the traction sutures to the forehead with Mastisol (Ferndale Labs, Ferndale, MI) and Steri-Strips (3M Health Care, St. Paul, MN) in both unilateral or bilateral cases. Unilateral cases may be patched with an oval eye pad. Ice is placed postoperatively for 15 minutes per hour for several hours. The traction sutures are removed at 24 to 48 hours. The 6-0 silk sutures with rubber band bolsters are removed at 10 to 12 days postoperatively.

COMPLICATIONS

The most common complication in upper or lower eyelid retraction repair is undercorrection.[2] It is important to overcorrect at various points to account for postoperative healing with the tendency for recurrent retraction. If this problem should become obvious with the upper lid early in the postoperative course, the author advises the patient to massage downward for 5 minutes several times a day while holding the brow in position. This procedure frequently is done incorrectly, and so it should be demonstrated to the patient carefully. The massage should be carried out for several weeks.

Persistent or recurrent retraction beyond this time will need to be addressed with a second procedure using the techniques already discussed but in a more aggressive fashion. Any scar bands will also have to be lysed. The author prefers to wait for approximately 3 months before performing this procedure to allow the original postoperative inflammation with concomitant increased tissue vascularization to abate. This will tend to promote a "cleaner" operative field with less hemorrhage and reduce the chances of significant scarring.

If persistent retraction following lower lid retraction repair is detected shortly after primary repair, several steps should be considered. If this situation becomes apparent within the first 24 to 48 hours, the upward traction suture will be tightened and left for up to a week. After a 3-month healing period, if the lid is still retracted, a second procedure will need to be performed with an interpositional spacer if one was not originally used. A secondary graft may need to be applied, with more overcorrection of the width of the spacer or possibly a change in spacer material (e.g., acellular dermis to ear cartilage).

Overcorrection of the upper lid will need to be addressed with a second procedure. This can be done with a standard levator advancement (see Chapter 6) or an internal (Muller's muscle–conjunctiva) resection (see Chapter 7). Lower lid overcorrection also needs to be corrected surgically.

Keratitis is generally caused by suture material, which the surgeon should find and remove. If this is not possible, copious lubricants or antibiotic ointment may be used until the material dissolves. A bandage soft contact lens may also be employed.

Occasionally in lower lid retraction repair, the spacer material will tend to shift or produce a prominent area of irregular healing, sometimes with color changes in the lid (representing the spacer material). A second surgery will generally need to be performed to remove the original spacer material and scar tissue.

Preseptal and orbital cellulitis are uncommon following these types of repair. Management of such infections is essentially identical to that in the unoperated patient. Mild to moderate cases of nonfebrile preseptal cellulitis should undergo Gram's stain and culture of any open or draining wound. Obvious abscesses should be drained. The patient should then be treated with a broad-spectrum oral antibiotic and followed closely.

Severe, febrile or toxic preseptal cellulitis or suspected cases of orbital cellulitis require immediate hospitalization with stain/culture, complete blood count, and blood cultures. Axial and coronal computed tomographic images of the orbit are made, and any obvious abscesses should be drained. The patient should then be treated with broad-spectrum antibiotics intravenously. An infectious disease consult may be appropriate.

REFERENCES

1. Stangler RA, Nesi FA, Valvo F. Complications of blepharoplasty. In: Nesi FA, Lisman RD, Levine MR, eds. *Smith's Ophthalmic and Plastic Reconstructive Surgery*. St Louis: Mosby-Year Book, 1998:436–447.

2. Karesh JW. Eyelid retraction: Evaluation, management and treatment. In: Mauriella JA Jr, ed. *Unfavorable Results of Eyelid and Lacrimal Surgery: Prevention and Management*. Boston: Butterworth-Heinemann Medical; 2000:275–305.

3. Baylis HI, Goldberg RA, Groth MJ. Complications of lower blepharoplasty. In: Putterman AM, ed. *Cosmetic Oculoplastic Surgery*. Philadelphia: WB Saunders; 1999:429–456.

4. Schwartz NG, Murphy M, Cohen MS. Lower eyelid retraction and cicatricial ectropion. In: Bosniak S, et al. *Principles and Practice of Ophthalmic Plastic and Reconstructive Surgery*. Philadelphia: WB Saunders; 1996:438–446.

5. Socket repair and reconstruction. In: Nesi FA, Gladstone GJ, Brazzo BG, et al, eds. *Ophthalmic and Facial Plastic Surgery: A Compendium of Reconstructive and Aesthetic Techniques*. Thorofare, NJ: Stack Incorporated; 2000:136–137.

13

Eyelid Tumor Excision and Reconstruction

• Taj G. Khan
• George O. Stasior
• Orkan George Stasior

Eyelid tumors must be evaluated carefully for proper diagnosis and treatment. Once a lesion has been identified, careful attention must be paid to clinical history, size, texture, margins, eyelash loss, color, vascularity, movability, and ulceration. For potentially malignant lesions, it is important to thoroughly palpate regional lymph nodes to check for local spread. This complete evaluation will help the surgeon develop a clinical index of suspicion that guides treatment.

EVALUATION

Common benign eyelid tumors include papillomas and seborrheic keratoses, both of which commonly occur with increasing frequency as patients age. Papillomas occur in both sessile and pedunculated forms and can be solitary or multiple. Seborrheic keratoses (Fig. 13.1) are discrete, movable, elevated, tan to brown lesions that have three histological variants: hyperacanthotic, acanthotic, and adenoid.[1] These tumors may be observed with photographic documentation and follow-up every 4 to 6 months. If these lesions become suspicious (i.e., increase in size, change in color, etc.) or bother the patient, surgical intervention by excisional biopsy with primary closure or adjacent tissue advancement is recommended. Full-thickness wedge resection may be considered for involvement of the eyelid margin and offers excellent cosmesis.

Molluscum contagiosum is a cutaneous pox virus that can infect the eyelids. Although frequently found in young healthy children, these lesions are being diagnosed with increasing frequency in patients with acquired immunodeficiency syndrome (AIDS).[2] Clinically, these elevated lesions are reddish-tan with a central umbilication and

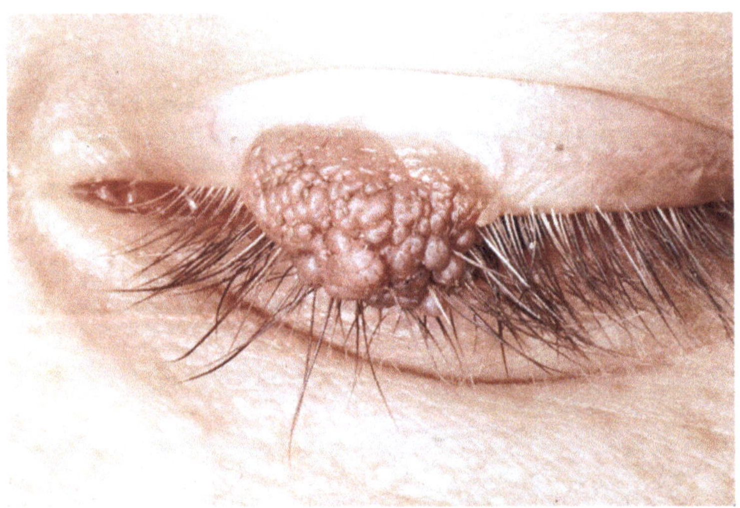

FIGURE 13.1. Seborrheic keratosis of the upper eyelid.

Eyelid Tumor Excision and Reconstruction

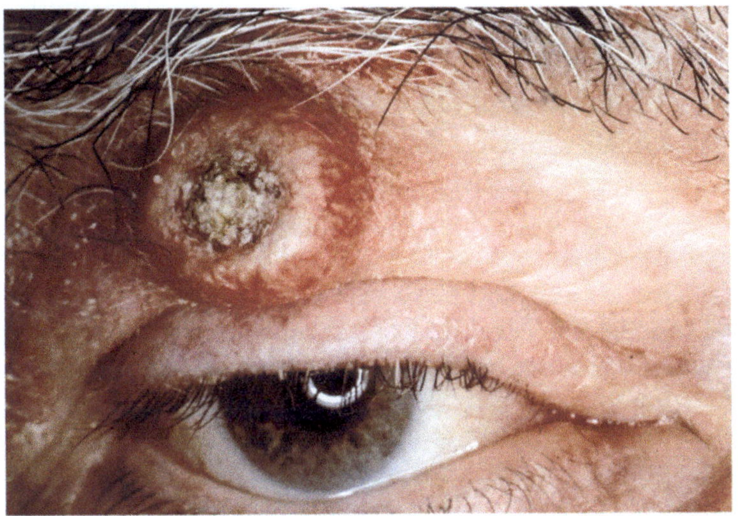

FIGURE 13.2. Classic keratoacanthoma with a central keratin core.

may spontaneously regress. Patients with eyelid margin involvement may present with a chronic follicular conjunctivitis as the virus sheds into the tear film. The recommended treatment includes excisional biopsy or cryotherapy.

Keratoacanthomas are benign, freely movable elevated lesions that rapidly grow. The tumor (Fig. 13.2) is similar in its clinical appearance to noduloulcerative basal cell carcinoma and displays well-differentiated squamous cells with a central keratin core. Histopathologically, this tumor is often confused with squamous cell carcinomas (SCC), and the pathologist requires the clinical history of "rapid growth" to make the proper diagnosis. Cryotherapy can be considered for smaller lesions after confirmatory biopsy. Although these tumors may spontaneously regress, the authors find that complete excision leads to the best cosmetic result.

Actinic keratoses are examples of premalignant eyelid tumors that are common in older Caucasian patients. Also known as "solar" or "senile keratoses," actinic keratoses occur as multiple sessile plaques in areas of sun-damaged skin. Actinic keratoses may undergo malignant transformation to squamous cell carcinoma. The recommended treatment is excisional biopsy.

Basal cell carcinomas (BCC) accounts for 90% of all malignant eyelid tumors. They most commonly occur in fair-skinned adults in the 50- to 80-year-old age group and affect the lower eyelid in approximately 50% of cases, followed by the medial canthus, upper eyelid, and lateral canthus in decreasing order of frequency.[3]

Subtypes of BCC include nodular (see later: Fig. 13.8A), noduloulcerative, cystic (Fig. 13.3), and morpheaform. The more common, less aggressive forms include the nodular and noduloulcerative types, which are firm, round, and have fine vascularity. Although most cystic eyelid lesions are benign, BCC can occur with cystic variation.[4] The less common, more aggressive form is the morpheaform or sclerosing type, which is pale, flat, and has indistinct margins. Histopathologically, this subtype sends fingerlike projections into clinically healthy tissue and may present with areas of eyelash loss (madarosis).

BCC has a histological spectrum, which ranges from nests of well-differentiated basal cells to poorly defined basal cells with variable dermal extension. If neglected or incompletely excised, BCC can have devastating results, with local and regional invasion to the globe, orbit, nasal cavity, and brain.

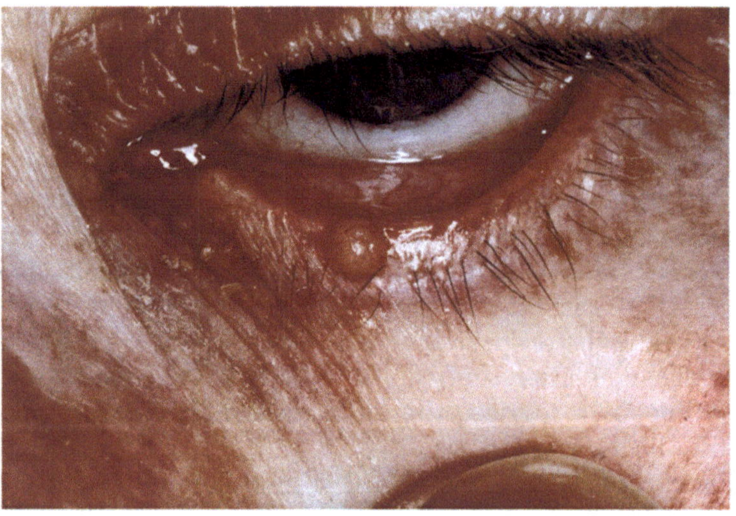

FIGURE 13.3. Cystic basal cell carcinoma, which appears as a benign lesion.

 Eyelid Tumor Excision and Reconstruction

The authors utilize excisional biopsy with frozen section monitoring to ensure clean margins of surrounding tissue. Biopsies of the tissue margins are performed and the pathologist reviews the specimens intraoperatively. The pathologist communicates with the surgeon, who carefully adjusts the surgical margins until the tumor has been completely excised.

Some authors advocate Mohs micrographic surgery as a useful treatment alternative once the malignancy of a tumor has been established by means of biopsy. This technique ensures high cure rates, minimizes recurrence, and allows a maximum preservation of normal tissue to facilitate eyelid reconstruction. Especially useful for excision of malignant tumors of the medial canthus, this process involves the sequential excision of malignant tissue with orientation of the specimen to anatomical landmarks. The tissue is then mapped according to unique color codes and processed to microscopically examine 100% of the tissue margins.[5] Although Mohs surgery affords several advantages, it is an expensive and time-consuming technique with limited availability.

Squamous cell carcinomas are the second most common type of malignant eyelid tumors, occurring in elderly, fair-skinned patients with a history of sun exposure. The in situ form is known as Bowen's disease, which appears as an erythematous, crusted, keratotic lesion.[6] Five clinical subtypes of SCC are nodular, papillomatous, cystic, placoid, and ulcerated.[1] Unlike BCC, SCC may display more aggressive behavior, with perineural spread and metastasis to regional lymph nodes.[7] The recommended treatment is excision with margins of at least 2 mm and deep tissues with frozen section monitoring. Lymph node dissection and biopsy may be necessary to stage this eyelid tumor. Although surgical excision is the most effective treatment, radiation and cryotherapy may be useful in special cases.

Sebaceous gland carcinomas (Fig. 13.4) comprise less than 5% of malignant eyelid tumors and are even more aggressive locally than BCC and SCC. Although more frequently seen with advancing age, these malignancies can arise in younger patients who have undergone orbital radiation therapy. Commonly arising on the upper eyelid and from the meibomian glands, sebaceous cell carcinomas present in nodular, diffuse, and pedunculated forms.[1] They have a yellow coloration with adjacent loss of cilia and can masquerade as chronic blepharitis or recurrent chalazia.

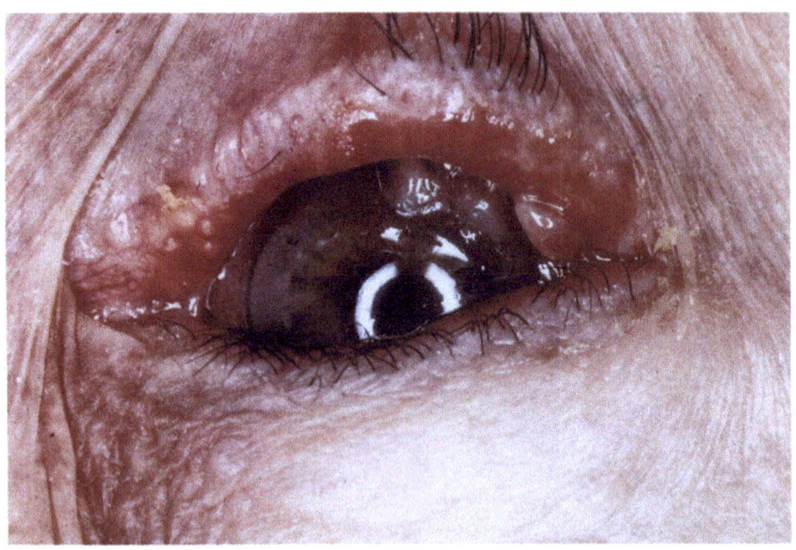

FIGURE 13.4. Diffuse form of sebaceous cell carcinoma with thickened eyelid margin and madarosis.

Recognition of pagetoid growth is an important distinguishing feature of these eyelid tumors. After confirmatory incisional biopsy,[8] excision with frozen section controls with at least 5 mm margins is recommended to reduce recurrence.[9] It is important for the surgeon to realize that sebaceous gland carcinoma is not always clearly identified with frozen section monitoring. These specimens may be transported in formaldehyde for special staining, including staining with Oil Red-O. Additionally, lipid stains must be performed *before* paraffin section preparation.[10]

Malignant melanomas (MM) are potentially lethal and comprise approximately 1% of malignant eyelid tumors. Primarily arising on sun-exposed areas of Caucasian patients of any age group, these tumors can appear as sessile or pedunculated lesions with or without ulceration. Four histological types are nodular (most common), superficial spreading, lentigo maligna, and acral lentiginous.[11] After confirmatory incisional biopsy, wide excision of normal skin has been proposed for malignant melanomas of the eyelid.[12] Sentinel lymph node mapping and biopsy can potentially assist in overall patient management.[13] Other treatment options not completely established

    Eyelid Tumor Excision and Reconstruction

include plaque radiotherapy,[14] cryotherapy, chemotherapy, and immunotherapy.[15]

Metastatic eyelid tumors account for less than 1% of malignant eyelid lesions. The most common primary sites include breast, gastrointestinal system, and respiratory system in descending order of frequency.[16]

Kaposi's sarcoma has become a major cause of morbidity and mortality in AIDS patients. Additionally, ocular adnexal involvement occurs in 20% of all AIDS patients with systemic Kaposi's sarcoma.[17]

Upper eyelid eversion is of tremendous importance in the evaluation of the eyelids. Malignant eyelid tumors, such as malignant melanoma (Fig. 13.5), may arise from the palpebral aspect of the conjunctiva and should not be overlooked.

It is important for the surgeon to develop a precise clinical index of suspicion by carefully evaluating the nature of the eyelid tumor. Incisional biopsies may be useful for confirmatory diagnosis of suspicious lesions and can dictate appropriate surgical planning. Frozen section monitoring with direct communication with the pathologist facilitates complete surgical excision. Once the tumor has been completely excised, the surgeon must evaluate the nature of the eyelid defect to plan for the appropriate reconstruction.

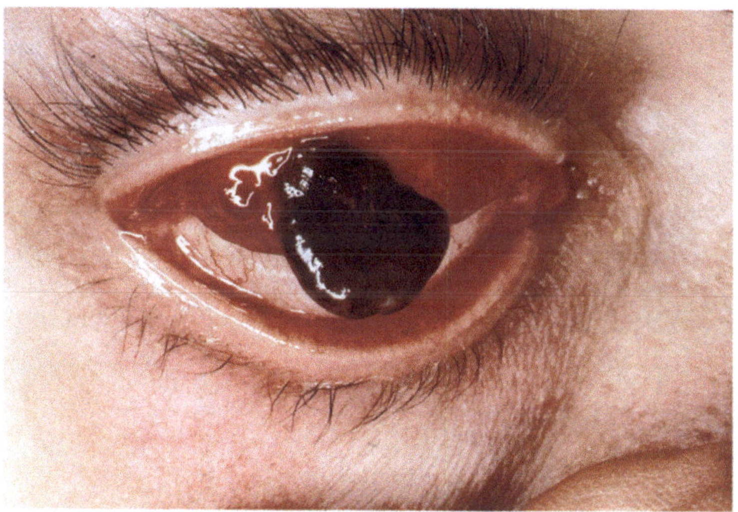

FIGURE 13.5. Conjunctival malignant melanoma.

Eyelid Reconstruction Principles

Restoration of eyelid function is predicated upon the principles of anatomy. Understanding this basic concept helps the surgeon to tailor technique and prevent complications before they occur. Total or subtotal lid defects cannot be closed primarily and require reconstruction of both the anterior and posterior lamellae.

The anterior lamella, consisting of skin and orbicularis muscle, receives its blood supply from the outer cutaneous layer. The posterior lamella, consisting of conjunctiva and tarsus, receives its blood supply from the conjunctival vasculature. Proper eyelid function provides a smooth inner mucosal surface in contact with the globe and structural support from the tarsal plate and canthal tendon attachments.

The choice of surgical reconstruction of the upper versus the lower eyelid depends upon the inherent functions of each. The upper lid must have vertical mobility and afford adequate corneal protection. Repair should be accomplished by providing a stable margin, smooth conjunctival surface, and functioning levator complex. The lower lid, which functions to facilitate the tear-pump mechanism, also should have both vertical and horizontal support to achieve apposition to the globe.

When reconstructing an eyelid, the surgeon must take into account the extent of the defect, its vascular supply, and the stability of both medial and lateral eyelid fixation. Eyelid defects not involving the lid margin can usually be closed with cutaneous or myocutaneous advancement flaps. In most patients, defects measuring one-quarter to one-third of the lid margin can be reconstructed with the aid of a lateral canthotomy and cantholysis. Defects involving more than one-third of the lid margin usually require additional reconstructive techniques.

The surgeon should also consider whether partial or total reconstruction of the anterior or posterior lamella might be required. It is essential to properly evaluate not only the quantity of the defect but also the type of tissue needed to reconstruct a properly functioning eyelid.

BASIC TECHNIQUES

Direct Closure of the Defect

Eyelid defects not involving the eyelid margin, but primarily involving the anterior lamella, can often be repaired by direct closure or by means of cutaneous or myocutaneous advancement flaps. Undermining of adjacent tissue is often necessary. Care should be taken not to distort the eyelid margin.

The surgeon must be careful not to cause eyelid malposition or conjuntivochalasis by placing too much tension on the wound. If these problems become evident during or after closure, a local skin flap, myocutaneous advancement flap, or full-thickness skin graft to release skin tension should help to resolve the condition.

Primary Eyelid Margin Closure

Defects from one-quarter to one-third of the lid margin usually can be closed primarily (Fig. 13.6). The cut ends of the eyelid margin should be reapproximated with minimal tension. Two or three double-armed 6-0 silk sutures are placed through corresponding margin landmarks and into the tarsal plate. These marginal sutures can be

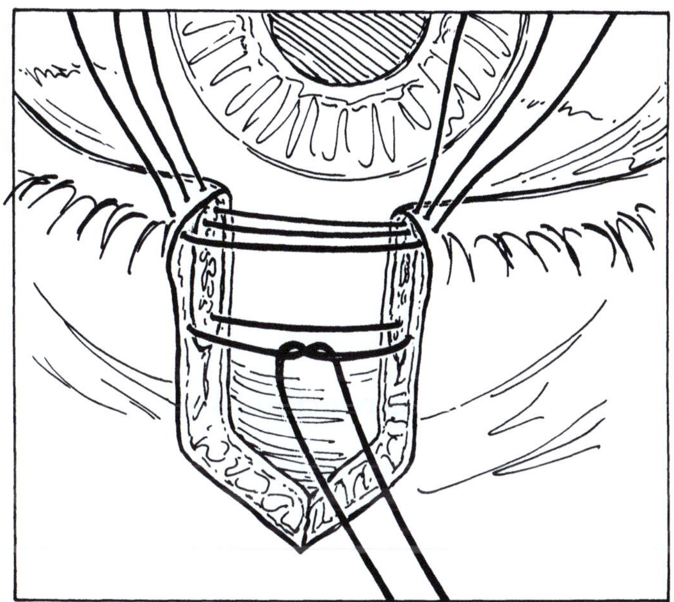

FIGURE 13.6. Classic three-suture technique for repair of margin lacerations. (Reproduced with permission from Classification and treatment of eyelid malposition. In: Nesi FA, Gladstone JG, Brazzo BG, et al., eds. *Ophthalmic and Facial Plastic Surgery: A Compendium of Aesthetic and Reconstructive Techniques.* Thorofare, NJ: Slack Incorporated, 2000:88.)

placed at the epidermal–mucosal junction, the gray line, and/or the eyelash margin. One or two interrupted 6-0 Vicryl sutures on spatulated needles are used to reappose the tarsal plate. Proper internal fixation and alignment of the tarsal plate are important in achieving a satisfactory result.

Common problems encountered in the healing period include "notching" at the lid margin, corneal abrasion from suture irritation, and poor wound eversion. The occurrence of these side effects can be reduced by properly aligning tarsus, eyelid margin, and eyelashes during closure. Conjunctiva must not be incorporated in tarsal sutures; otherwise the suture will abrade the eye. Also, if sutures are placed too posteriorly at the lid margin, they will cause abrasions. Careful placement of a "far-far/near-near" vertical mattress suture at the eyelid margin can ensure proper tension and alignment.

During closure, the surgeon may notice that too much horizontal tension is placed on the wound. To reduce the possibility of wound dehiscence or pronounced scar formation, the surgeon should perform 5 to 7 mm canthotomy, as described in Chapter 10 (see Fig. 10.3) through the skin and orbicularis muscle in the lateral canthal angle. This step usually needs to be followed by a cantholysis (see Fig. 10.4) to disinsert the inferior crus of the lateral canthal tendon from the orbital rim and the lateral lower eyelid retractors from the periosteum. This technique allows the lateral eyelid margin to be mobilized medially approximately 3 to 5 mm. Absorbable sutures can be used in reapposing the lateral canthal angle.

ADVANCED TECHNIQUES

Lower Eyelid Reconstruction, Anterior Lamella

Myocutaneous Advancement Flaps
Advancement flaps afford a good match of tissue color and texture. Anterior lamellar defects greater than one-third of the lid margin can be managed with a myocutaneous cheek rotation popularized by Imre and Tenzel (Fig. 13.7), a semicircular advancement flap popularized by Mustarde (discussed later under Upper Eyelid Reconstruction: see Fig. 13.9), or a composite tissue graft.[18,19]

Several complications are commonly encountered with these techniques. Lateral canthal deformity, with thinning and rounding of the lateral canthal angle, is common. Reducing the horizontal tension (with canthotomy and cantholysis) will help to alleviate this deformity. Also, placement of a lateral canthal appositional suture, as pop-

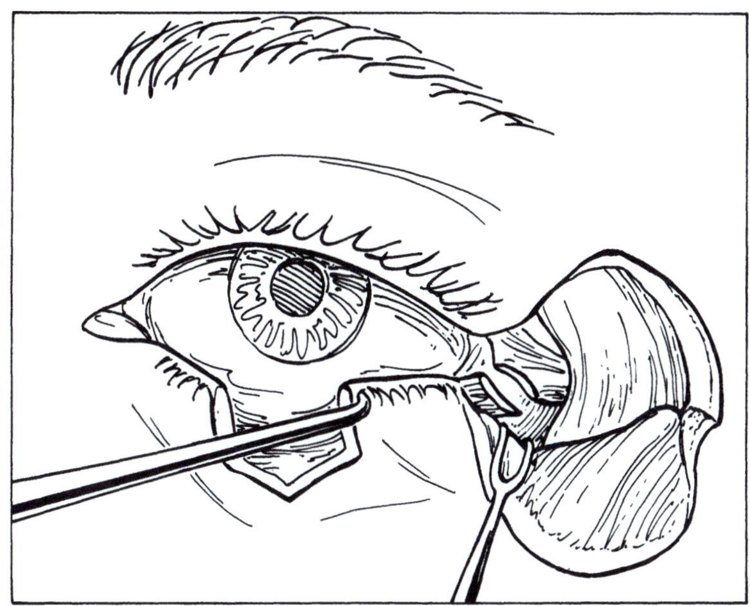

FIGURE 13.7. Semicircular temporal advancement flap. Following mass excision and incision of lateral canthal tendon, the skin–muscle flap is mobilized. (Reproduced with permission from the illustrator Virginia Cantarella, and from Eyelid reconstruction. In: Nesi FA, Waltz KL, eds. *Smith's Practical Techniques in Ophthalmic Plastic Surgery*. St. Louis: Mosby-Year Book; 1994:73.)

ularized by Dortzbach, may be useful. This step is performed by placing a buried absorbable suture to align the upper and lower lid margins at the lateral commissure before closure of the skin and muscle.

As healing occurs, lid retraction and ectropion may develop. The surgeon should remember to minimize vertical tension by making the vertical dimension of the flap greater than the horizontal dimension. During healing, the lower lid margin should rest above the inferior corneal limbus, which may require temporary placement of traction sutures or tarsorraphy.

Lid margin instability can lead to cicatricial ectropion or entropion. This outcome can be eliminated if smaller and thinner advancement flaps, which reduce vertical tension and provide margin stability, are developed. Postoperative cicatrix can be excised and repaired with tarsoconjunctival graft (for posterior lamellar scar) or skin graft (for anterior lamellar scar).

Free Full-Thickness Skin Graft (FTSG)
Recipient sites for skin grafts must be evaluated under mild tension. The graft should mold to the contour of the deep eyelid struc-

tures. A template is useful to measure proper graft size. Donor sites are chosen on the basis of skin thickness, color, texture, and the lack of hair follicles. Optimal donor sites in order of preference include adjacent or opposite eyelid and posterior auricular, supraclavicular, and periaxillary skin. Upper or lower eyelid skin defects are best reconstructed with contralateral eyelid or postauricular skin. Atraumatic thinning of the graft is aesthetically important. Split-thickness skin grafts are occasionally used in severe burn victims when adequate full-thickness skin is not available.

Eyelid contracture secondary to small graft size and minimal dermis may compromise surgical outcome. The surgeon must remember to carefully assess the graft size with the defect under mild tension, allowing for adequate tissue to mold to the lid contour. Postoperatively, massage can be performed with application of firm pressure to the graft against underlying bone; if this fails, regrafting may be necessary.

As indicated in Chapter 10, some grafts demonstrate poor color and texture match (see Fig. 10.11). To reduce the chance of this occurring, the surgeon should atraumatically thin the FTSG down to the rete pegs. It is important to note that dermal collagen continues to change for at least 6 months after reconstruction, causing anatomical alterations during that time.

To reduce the risk of graft necrosis, the surgeon must pay careful attention to the graft bed, which should be dry, uncharred, and well vascularized. Placement of small fenestrations ("pie crusting") and application of adequate pressure with bolsters such as dental sponges will reduce the risk of hematoma postoperatively.

Lower Eyelid Reconstruction, Posterior Lamella

Tarsoconjunctival Advancement Flap (Modified Hughes Procedure)

A two-stage reconstruction creates a smooth conjunctival surface and provides stability of the lower lid margin.[20] The tumor (Fig. 13.8A) is excised with frozen section monitoring. The amount of grafted tissue needed is determined by measuring the defect under tension.

An incision is made through the palpebral tarsus 4 mm from the upper eyelid margin with the lid everted over a Desmarres retractor. A tarsoconjunctival graft is then harvested with careful dissection of conjunctiva from Muller's muscle superiorly to decrease retraction of the donor site (Fig. 13.8B). The inferior edge of the tarsoconjunctival

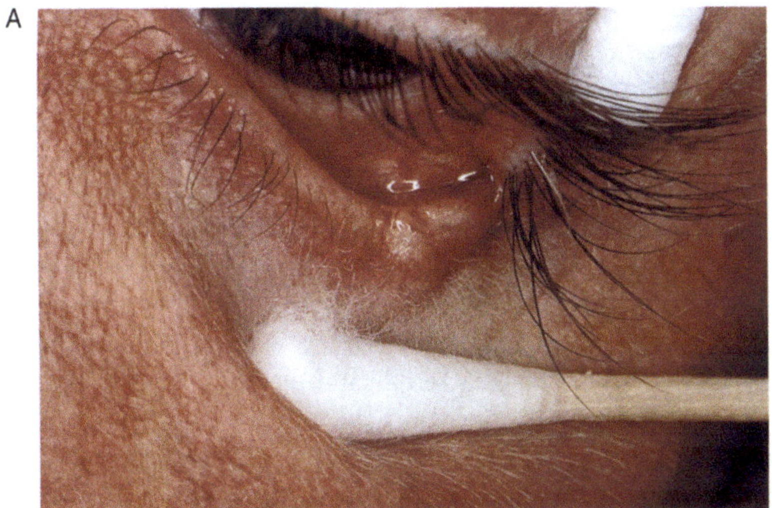

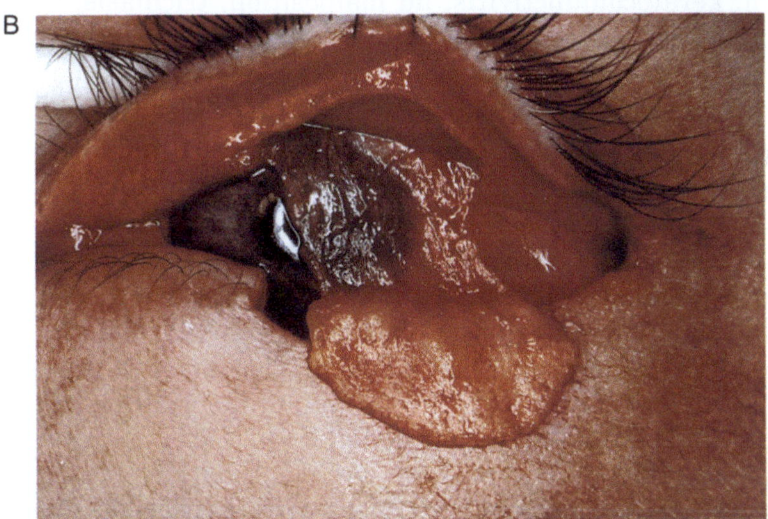

FIGURE 13.8. Modified Hughes procedure. (A) Preoperative 33-year-old patient with a nodular basal cell carcinoma of the left lower eyelid; full-thickness resection resulted in greater than 50% of lower eyelid deficit. (B) A tarsoconjunctival graft is harvested with sufficient superior dissection of conjunctiva from Muller's muscle to allow the graft to hang freely.

graft is sutured either to the conjunctiva of the remaining part of the lower eyelid or to conjunctiva advanced from the inferior fornix. The superior edge of the tarsal flap is placed 1 to 2 mm above the adjacent lower lid margin, "dovetailing" the graft into the recipient lid margin.

The anterior lamella is reconstructed by a myocutaneous advancement flap (Fig. 13.8C) or a full-thickness skin graft from the contralateral upper eyelid or postauricular region. Postoperatively, the advanced conjunctiva will thicken as it transitions into lower eyelid tissue.

Two to 4 weeks later, the second stage is completed with a tarsotomy and releasing of the grafted tissue from the upper eyelid (Fig. 13.8D). It is important to maintain lid margin integrity by beveling the incision anteriorly to create a higher posterior lamella. If necessary, additional canthal reconstruction is undertaken at this time.

Often, keratoconjunctivitis, lid malposition, trichiasis, and lacrimal pump palsy are noted after this reconstruction. The cause may be secondary to excess lower lid laxity. These conditions may be prevented if the surgeon remembers to transplant less tissue than the apparent size of the initial defect. Postoperatively, horizontal shortening of the lateral lower lid can alleviate this condition. Keratoconjunctivitis can be due to upper eyelid retraction, lid margin keratinization, trichiasis, distichiasis, and lanugo hairs.

Posterior lamellar keratinization and entropion are both treated by separation of the anterior and posterior lamellae, and recession of the anterior lamella of the lower eyelid. The lamellae are then secured with mattress sutures. Mucous membrane grafting can be performed to augment the posterior lamella.

Ectropion may be observed in several situations. If significant lower eyelid laxity is present, treatment with horizontally shortening (i.e., lateral tarsal strip: see Chapter 10) should be effective. Cicatricial ectropion can be improved by separating the anterior and posterior lamellae of the lower eyelid and advancing the anterior lamella superiorly. The lamellae are then secured with horizontal mattress sutures through the entire eyelid.

The incidence of lower eyelid retraction can be reduced if the surgeon divides the advancement flap 1 to 2 mm above the contralateral lower lid margin. The advancement flap pedicle must be trimmed flush with the upper lid tarsus to release all tension within the pedicle. Postoperative management of lid retraction requires advancement

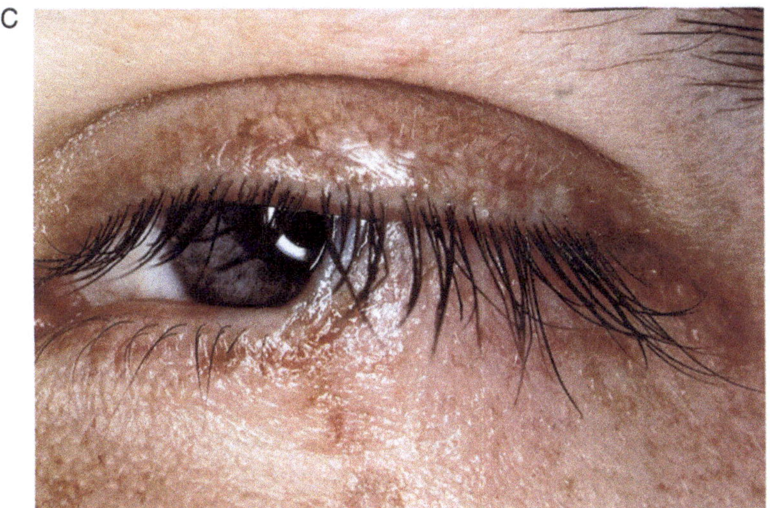

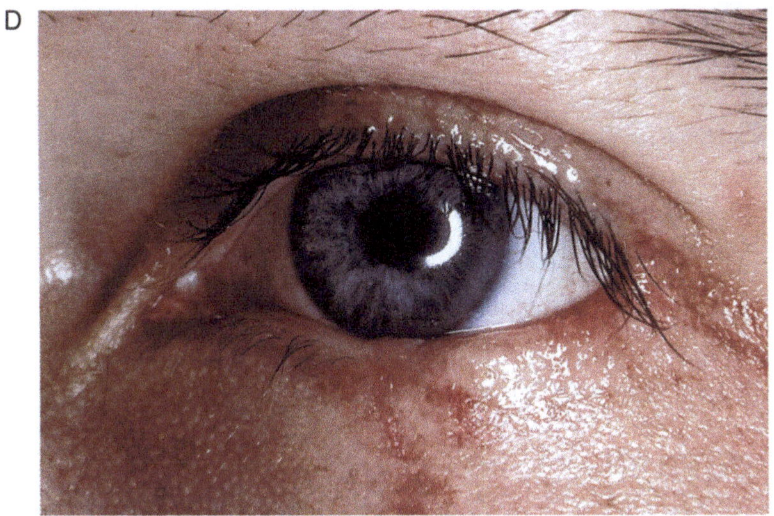

FIGURE 13.8. (C) The anterior lamella is reconstructed with a myocutaneous advancement flap. (D) Four weeks later, the second stage is completed with a tarsotomy and, if necessary, reconstruction of the lower eyelid margin.

of the posterior lamella or an additional tarsoconjunctival graft with anterior lamellar revision, including local flaps or FTSG.

Lower eyelid margin notching can be avoided if the surgeon carefully places sutures and avoids excessive horizontal tension. Postoperatively, excess tissue adjacent to the notch may be trimmed or cauterized. In cases of excess lid laxity, the notch can be excised and the edges reapposed.

Frequently, retraction of the donor (upper) eyelid forms after the advancement flap is severed. During the initial procedure, adequate conjunctiva and Muller's muscle must be mobilized. Meticulous dissection of Muller's muscle from the conjunctiva can be facilitated by ballooning the conjunctiva with a local anesthetic mixed with epinephrine. Additionally, it is important to perform adequate conjunctival dissection superiorly to prevent excess tension on the tarsoconjunctival graft. Postoperative treatment of retraction includes a tarsotomy and recession of posterior lamella with a tissue spacer if necessary.

Tarsoconjunctival Transposition Flap (Hewes Flap)

A tarsoconjunctival transposition flap is an important alternative to the Hughes procedure. A lateral flap is developed to reconstruct a large, full-thickness posterior lamellar defect, providing blood supply, marginal stability, and satisfactory cosmesis. This procedure is particularly beneficial to the monocular patient who will maintain sight in the eye postoperatively.[21] However, this is a somewhat less desirable alternative because of possible lateral canthal deformity, donor site retraction, and disruption of lacrimal gland tubules.

Composite Grafts

Composite grafts, which involve multiple layers of the eyelid, are becoming a preferred method of posterior eyelid reconstruction.[22] After a graft has been harvested, part of the anterior lamella is removed, and the remaining margin and posterior lamella are sutured into the defect. The anterior lamella is reconstructed with a cutaneous or myocutaneous advancement flap. These grafts may be harvested from the ipsilateral or contralateral lid, and a large defect extending over more than half the lid can be reconstructed by sewing multiple composite free grafts together.

Marginal notching can occur at donor or recipient sites. This problem can be prevented by meticulous margin realignment and avoiding excess horizontal tension. Although madarosis will often occur, the eyelashes tend to regrow within a few months, but are usually

		Eyelid Tumor Excision and Reconstruction

finer, shorter, and hypopigmented. If necrosis occurs, debridement should be performed initially. If necessary, and if the blood supply is intact, a pedicle flap can be mobilized.

Mucous Membrane Grafts

Mucous membrane grafts are used in posterior lamellar reconstruction to restore a smooth lid surface against the globe. Buccal mucosa is a common source for this type of graft. During harvesting, the surgeon should place a suture on the anterior mucosal surface to maintain correct orientation, thereby avoiding burying of the epithelial surface. Proper illumination and adequate exposure will help the surgeon to minimize donor site complications. The wound may be closed with 4-0 plain gut suture, or it may be allowed to granulate. If the graft is placed under minimal tension, the risk of keratoconjunctivitis and graft hypertrophy will be reduced.

Free Cartilage Grafts

Cartilage grafts restore stability and rigidity to the lid margin and thereby reduce postoperative contracture.[23] Common harvesting sites include the palatine and auricular regions. The hard palate free graft is harvested from the roof of the mouth and is composed of a mucous membrane surface and a deep layer of dense connective tissue. The incision size is approximately 5×25 mm^2 and has an anteroposterior orientation off the midline of the hard palate. The donor site is left to heal by primary intention or can be protected with a prefit impression plate. This graft is carefully thinned to 1 mm. The surgeon should measure 1 to 2 mm of hard palate for each millimeter of vertical deficit and orient the mucosal side of the graft toward the globe.

When there is remaining tarsal plate, the tarsus should be used to reconstruct the lid margin; otherwise, the palatine graft may be used. In the lower eyelid, the surgeon reapproximates the margins of the graft with buried absorbable sutures. A dissolvable bandage contact lens is placed over the cornea for the first 48 hours, and a horizontal traction suture is placed to support the lower eyelid for the first postoperative week.

Common complications include keratoconjunctivitis secondary to keratinization, suture erosion, and exposure. The surgeon can reduce the incidence of these events by using partial-thickness bites with a spatulated needle and placing a bandage contact lens. To reduce bleeding, the peripheral vascular arcades should be avoided. Judicious use of cautery, thrombin, and modified collagen (Avitene, Superstat) can assist in limiting bleeding from palatine bed.[24,25]

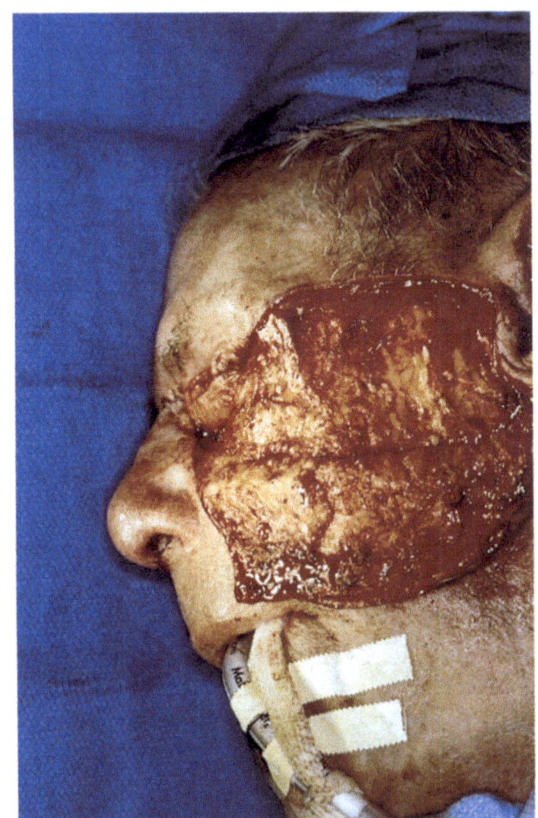

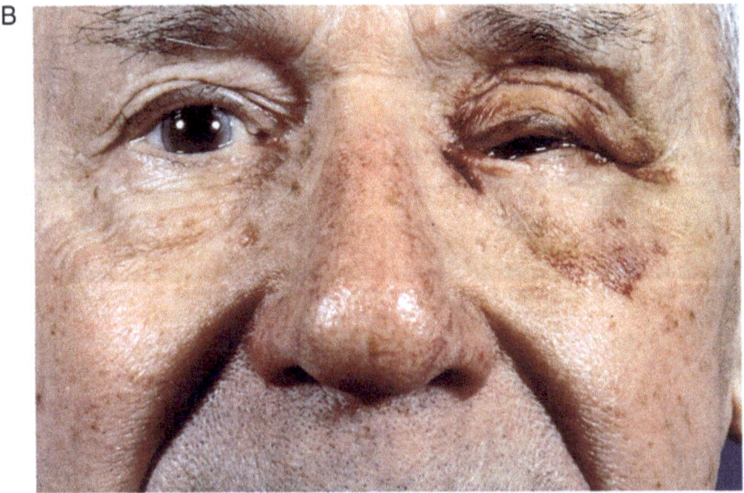

FIGURE 13.9. Mustarde-type rotation flap. (A) Intraoperative view. (B) Following exenteration for invasive basal cell carcinoma and orbital reconstruction, a Mustarde flap was used to reconstruct the upper and lower eyelids. (Courtesy of Ian T. Jackson, M.D.)

Upper Eyelid Reconstruction

Full-Thickness Rotation Flap from Lower Lid (Mustarde Flap)

A large Mustarde rotation flap (Fig. 13.9) can be used to treat upper lid defects of various sizes with a medially or laterally based full-thickness rotation from the lower eyelid.[19] The surgeon must allow for adequate blood supply by avoiding excessive tension.

Lower Eyelid Full-Thickness Advancement Flap (Cutler–Beard Flap)

A Cutler–Beard flap is employed to reconstruct large upper eyelid defects (half or more of the horizontal length). This technique (Fig. 13.10) involves a lower lid full-thickness myocutaneous advancement flap advanced under a marginal bridge.[26] A full-thickness lower eye-

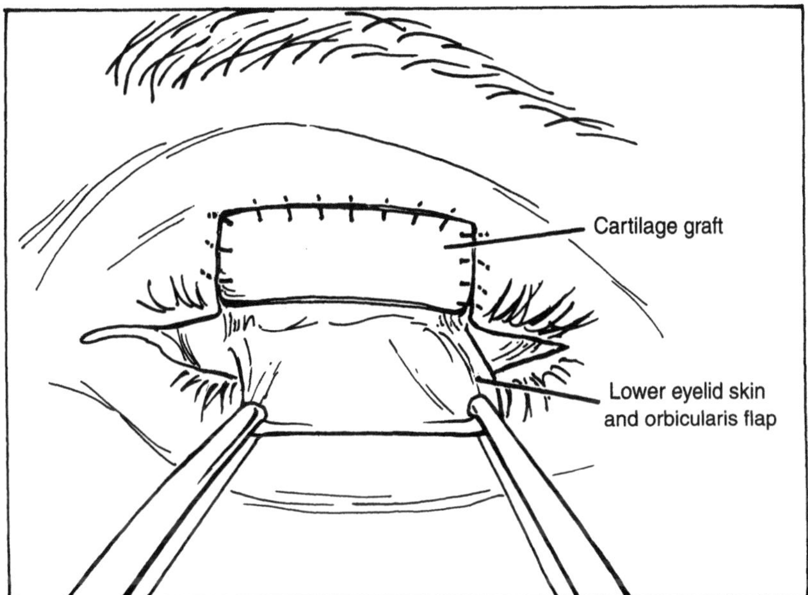

FIGURE 13.10. Lower eyelid full-thickness advancement flap. Following mass excision and development of advancement flap, the conjunctival layer is repaired. A cartilage graft may be sutured to provide stability to the lid, then the skin layers are closed. (Reproduced with permission from the illustrator, Virginia Cantarella, and from Eyelid reconstruction. In: Nesi FA, Waltz KL, eds. *Smith's Practical Techniques in Ophthalmic Plastic Surgery*. St. Louis: Mosby-Year Book; 1994:79.)

lid flap is developed 5 to 6 mm below the lower eyelid margin. A lower lid margin bridge with its own vascular supply is formed. The posterior lamella of the new upper eyelid margin can be stabilized by reconstruction with either banked sclera or ear cartilage.

Second-stage flap separation should not be performed until at least 6 to 8 weeks later to allow for peripheral vascular ingrowth and adequate time for contracture of the pedicle as it heals. Premature graft separation may lead to graft failure and eyelid contraction. At the time of separation, it is important to overcorrect the amount of mucous membrane left behind and to shorten the anterior lamella relative to the posterior lamella with a beveled incision to prevent both eyelid contraction and internal keratinization of the eyelid margin.

Rigidity and poor mobility of the upper lid can lead to lagophthalmos and ptosis. To prevent these complications, a three-layered reconstruction (conjunctiva, cartilage, and skin) should be considered. This technique also secures the levator to the upper aspect of the cartilage graft to improve upper lid mobility. Additionally, creation of an advancement flap 6 to 8 mm below the lower lid margin will decrease lower eyelid retraction.

Upper eyelid retraction with exposure keratopathy can occur if scarring occurs at any level. The surgeon should consider dissection of cicatricial tissue, advancement of posterior lamella, and suturing an FTSG to the upper lid.

Margin instability leads to ectropion or entropion, and resultant keratoconjunctivitis. This undesirable result can be prevented by stabilizing the anterior and posterior lamellae in relation to each other with through-and-through absorbable sutures at the second stage. Postoperative entropion can be managed with anterior lamellar recession with mucous membrane grafting (i.e., buccal mucosa), a free tarsoconjunctival composite graft from the contralateral upper lid, or scleral graft spacers to enhance margin stability.

Necrosis of the bridge at the donor site may result from disruption of the tarsus or marginal arcade of the lower lid during initial reconstruction. Cold compresses, pressure patching, and placement of sutures into the bridge predispose to vascular compromise. The author recommends excising necrotic tissue and reanastomosing the bridge remnants. If insufficient tissue remains, the lower lid may be reconstructed with a Tenzel semicircular flap.

Transconjunctival Lower Lid Advancement Flap (Leone Flap)

The Leone flap is similar to a reverse modified Hughes procedure used in lower lid reconstruction.[27] A lower eyelid tarsal incision is fashioned 1.5 mm from the posterior lid margin and the conjunctiva is separated from the lower lid retractors. The tarsoconjunctival flap is then advanced and positioned into the upper lid defect with tarsus at the reconstructed margin. The anterior lamella is reconstructed with a cutaneous or myocutaneous graft. This reconstructive procedure provides posterior lamellar stability of the upper and lower eyelids combined with a smooth conjunctival surface.

Complications of this procedure and their management are similar to those described for the modified Hughes operation for lower lid reconstruction. In addition, there may be problems with upper lid mobility or the level of the lid margin, resulting in ptosis or upper lid retraction. Correction of these complications often requires levator surgery.

Sliding Tarsoconjunctival Flap

A sliding tarsoconjunctival flap allows repair of the posterior lamella of the upper eyelid. After careful dissection of Muller's muscle, a fornix-based tarsoconjunctival flap is transposed medially or laterally into the adjacent defect, thereby reconstructing the posterior lamella. The anterior lamella is then reconstructed with either an FTSG or an adjacent myocutaneous flap.

Medial Canthal Reconstruction

Spontaneous granulation has been a satisfactory and historically proven reconstructive alternative for medial canthus repair. A well-vascularized medial canthus is an excellent recipient bed for an FTSG harvested from an adjacent eyelid or posterior auricular region. These grafts offer an excellent color and texture match with minimal contraction (Fig. 13.11).

Deep internal fixation is required for reconstruction of the medial canthus. If medial fixation is absent, then transnasal wiring or microplating techniques can be utilized. If the posterior lacrimal crest is intact, a nonabsorbable posterior fixation suture with slight overcorrection can be used. This technique for reconstructing the posterior limb of the medial canthal ligament affords medial eyelid apposition to the globe and prevents pooling of tears and lacrimal pump dysfunction.

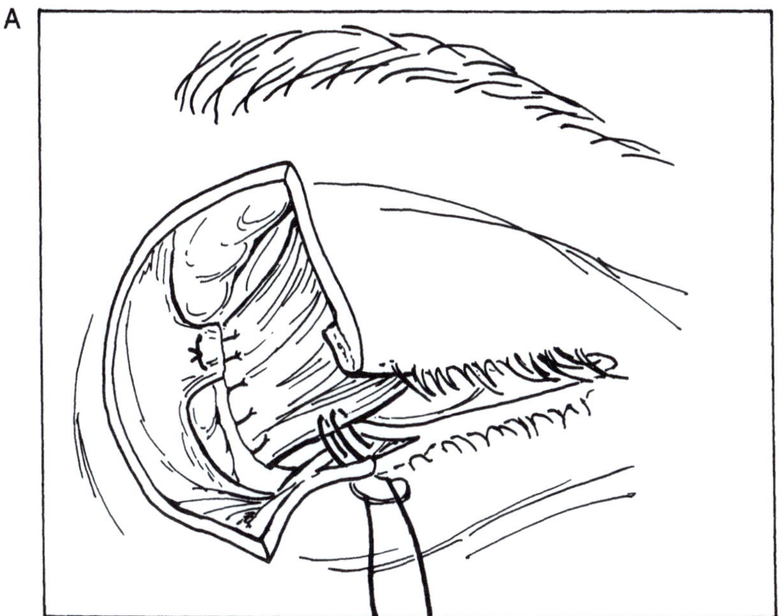

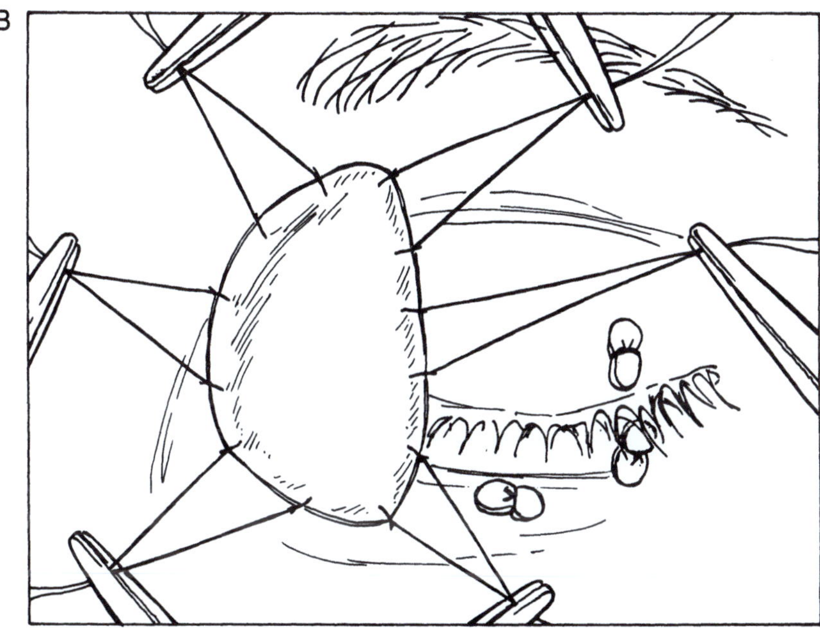

FIGURE 13.11. Medial canthal reconstruction. (A) Following mass excision, a tarsoconjunctival flap is transposed and sutured into position. The stump of the medial canthal tendon is sutured to the flap. (B) Free skin graft is placed over the defect. (Reproduced with permission from the illustrator, Virginia Cantarella, and from Eyelid reconstruction. In: Nesi FA, Waltz KL, eds. *Smith's Practical Techniques in Ophthalmic Plastic Surgery*. St. Louis: Mosby-Year Book; 1994:99–101.

Medial canthal reconstruction can be performed by a cutaneous or myocutaneous midline forehead flap (MFF)[28] (Fig. 13.12). The MFF is a useful way of using a well-vascularized pedicle flap to cover large medial canthal defects. The pedicle flap, based on the supratrochlear and supraorbital arteries, may extend up to 6 to 7 cm in length with a base of 3.0 to 3.5 cm. Second-stage reconstruction can take place as early as 3 weeks. To assess flap viability, the surgeon can utilize the "tourniquet" compression technique prior to division.

Complications of the MFF include excessively thick donor tissue and medial canthal angle deformity that may require a third-stage reconstruction. Other complications include distal flap necrosis and poor color/texture match.

Medial canthal reconstruction by any means may be complicated in the postoperative period by webbing, which can often be corrected with an epicanthal Z-plasty or a Y-V-plasty.[29] Double Z-plasties are particularly useful because they change the lines of tension and elon-

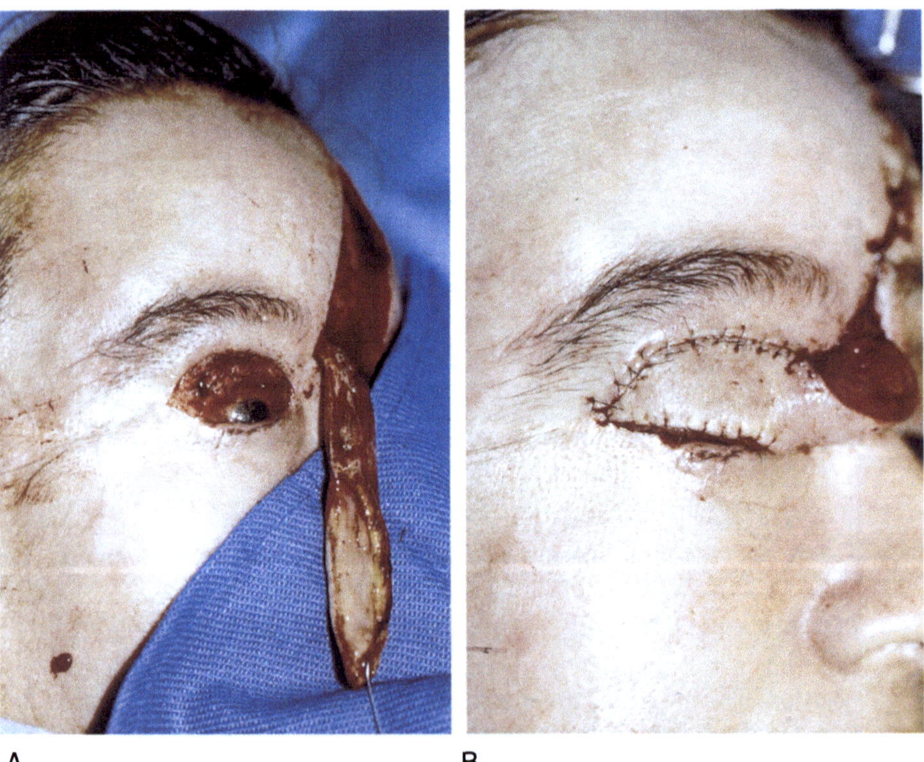

A   B

FIGURE 13.12. Midline forehead flap. (A) The forehead flap was lined with buccal mucosa 2 weeks earlier. (B) Total upper eyelid reconstruction, with flap sutured to skin and levator. (Courtesy of Ian T. Jackson, M.D.)

gate the tissue along the centralized "Z" limb. Proper intraoperative mapping is essential for meticulous medial canthal reconstruction.

Lateral Canthal Reconstruction

Reconstruction of the lateral canthus requires internal orbital fixation, adequate blood supply, fornix restoration, and a cutaneous cover. Lateral-based tarsoconjunctival transposition flaps can be used for large lower eyelid defects that extend into the lateral canthus (Fig. 13.13), with full-thickness skin grafts or advancement flaps developed for anterior lamellar reconstruction. When no lateral canthal tendon is present, the canthus can be reconstructed with a strip of periosteum based 3 to 5 mm inside the lateral orbital rim. If periosteum is lacking, holes can be drilled inside the lateral orbital rim to fixate a new lateral canthus with sutures, wires, or fascia (fascia lata or temporalis fascia).

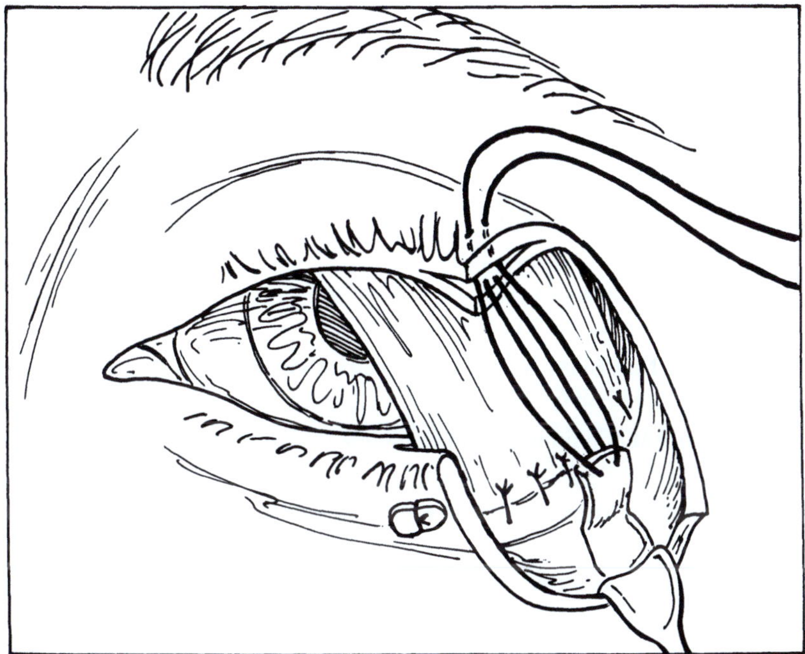

FIGURE 13.13. Lateral canthal reconstruction. After mass has been removed, a tarsoconjunctival flap is sutured into the defect. A periosteal hinged flap is created and sutured to the upper lid to recreate the canthal tendon. (Reproduced with permission from the illustrator, Virginia Cantarella, and from Eyelid reconstruction. In: Nesi FA, Waltz KL, eds. *Smith's Practical Techniques in Ophthalmic Plastic Surgery.* St. Louis: Mosby-Year Book; 1994:95.

Posterior fixation at Whitnall's tubercle provides good apposition of the lateral eyelid to the globe, and proper vertical placement of the angle is important to avoid canthal dystopia. Additionally, care must be taken to avoid suture placement too anteriorly on Whitnall's tubercle, which may cause a gap between the lateral lid and globe, leading to tear pooling and lacrimal pump dysfunction. Restoration of a smooth internal surface and adequate pocket in the lateral fornix will decrease adhesions and symblepharon. This may require free mucous membrane grafting and placement of a symblepharon ring or shell in the early postoperative period.

REFERENCES

1. Shields JA, Shields CL. *Eyelid and Conjunctival Tumors*. Philadelphia: Lippincott Williams & Wilkins; 1999:6,32,40.

2. Robinson MR, Udell IJ, Garber PF, et al. Molluscum contagiosum of the eyelids in patients with acquired immunodeficiency syndrome. *Ophthalmology* 1992;99:1745–1747.

3. Shields CL. Basal cell carcinoma of the eyelids. *Int Ophthalmol Clin* 1993;33:1–4.

4. Karciouglu ZA, Al-Hussain H, Svedberg AH. Cystic basal cell carcinoma of the eyelids. *Ophthalmic Plast Reconstr Surg* 1998;14:134–140.

5. Larson PO, et al. Mohs micrographic surgery for tumor excision. In: Albert DM, ed. *Ophthalmic Surgery: Principles and Techniques*. Malden, MA: Blackwell Science Publishers; 1999:1342.

6. Scott KR, Kronish JW. Premalignant lesions and squamous cell carcinoma. In: Albert DM, Jakobiec FA, eds. *Principles and Practice of Ophthalmology*. Philadelphia: Saunders; 1994:1734–1737.

7. Reifler DM, Hornblass A. Squamous cell carcinoma of the eyelid. *Survey Ophthalmol* 1986:349–365.

8. Putterman AM. Conjunctival map biopsy to determine pagetoid spread. *Am J Ophthalmol* 1968;102:87–90.

9. Dogru M, et al. Management of eyelid sebaceous carcinomas. *Ophthalmolgica* 1997;211:40–43.

10. Personal communication with ophthalmic pathologist Martha Farber, MD.

11. Grossniklaus HE, McLean IW. Cutaneous melanoma of the eyelid. *Ophthalmology* 1991;98:1867–1873.

12. Zoltie N, O'Neill TJ. Malignant melanomas of eyelid skin. *Plast Reconstr Surg* June 1989;83(6):994–996.

13. Esmaeli B, Eicher S, Delpassand E. Sentinel lymph node localization and biopsy for conjunctival melanomas. Presented at the Annual Scientific Symposium of the American Society of Ophthalmic Plastic and Reconstructive Surgery. Fall 2000; Dallas, TX.

14. Stanowsky A, Krey HF, Kopp J, et al. Irradiation of malignant eyelid melanoma with iodine-125 plaque. *Am J Ophthalmol* 1990;110:44–48.

15. Stannard CE. Malignant melanoma of the eyelid and palpebral conjunctiva treated with iodine-125 brachytherapy. *Ophthalmology* 2000;107(5):951–958.

16. Mansour AM, Hidayat AA. Metastatic eyelid disease. *Ophthalmology* 1987;94:667–670.

17. Dugel PU, Parkash SG. Frangieh GT. Ocular adenexal Kaposi's sarcoma in acquired immunodeficiency syndrome. *Am J Ophthalmol* 1990;110:500–503.

18. Tenzel RR. Reconstruction of the central one half of an eyelid. *Arch Ophthalmol* 1975;93:125–126.

19. Mustarde JC. *Repair and Reconstruction in the Orbital Region.* New York: Churchhill Livingstone; 1991:29,57–62,77–94.

20. Hughes WL. *Reconstructive Surgery of the Lids.* 2d ed. St Louis: Mosby; 1954:17,20–32,43–59,73–102,117–125,135–226.

21. Hewes EH, Sullivan JH, Beard C. Lower eyelid reconstruction by tarsal transposition. *Am J Ophthalmol* 1976;81:512–514.

22. Callahan A. Free composite eyelid graft. *Arch Ophthalmol* 1951;45:539–545.

23. Cohen MS, Shorr N. Eyelid reconstruction with hard palate mucosal grafts. *Ophthalmic Plast Reconstr Surg* 1992;8(3):183–195.

24. Tse DT, McCafferty LR. Controlled tissue expansion in periocular reconstructive surgery. *Ophthalmology* 1993;100:260–268.

25. Foster JA, Scheiner AJ, Wulc AE, et al. Intraoperative tissue expansion in eyelid reconstruction. *Ophthalmology* 1998;105:170–175.

26. Cutler NL, Beard C. A method for partial and total upper eyelid reconstruction. *Am J Ophthalmol* 1955;39:1–7.

27. Leone CR, Jr. Tarsoconjunctival advancement flaps for upper eyelid reconstruction. *Arch Ophthalmol* 1983;101:945–948.

28. Dortzbach RK, Hawes MJ. Midline forehead flap in reconstructive procedures of the lids and exenterated socket. *Ophthalmic Surg* 1981;12(4):257–268.

29. Hughes WL. Surgical treatment of congenital palpebral phimosis: the Y-V operation. *Arch Ophthalmol* 1955;54:586–590.

BIBLIOGRAPHY

Albert DM, ed. *Ophthalmic Surgery: Principles and Techniques.* Malden, MA: Blackwell Science Publishers; 1999:1364–1373.

Dortzbach RK. *Ophthalmic Plastic Surgery: Prevention and Management of Complications.* New York: Raven Press; 1994:125–140.

14

EXTERNAL DACRYOCYSTORHINOSTOMY

* Briggs E. Cook, Jr.
* Mark J. Lucarelli
* Bradley N. Lemke

The first steps to the successful management of a patient with a lacrimal disorder are obtaining an accurate history and performing a thorough clinical evaluation. A thorough evaluation usually leads to a correct diagnosis, which in turn leads to a high success rate. With an adequate anatomical foundation, the surgeon can increase the chance of success of dacryocystorhinostomy (DCR) surgery.

ANATOMICAL CORRELATION

The bony nose is formed by the frontonasal process. The nasal cavity is bisected anteriorly by the cartilaginous septum, which joins the vomer, a bony vertical plate of the ethmoid, posteriorly. Laterally, the nasal wall is thrown into three or more horizontal ridges termed turbinates, with a corresponding meatus below each turbinate (Fig. 14.1).

The inferior turbinate arises from the medial wall of the maxillary sinus and is the largest of the turbinates. The progressively smaller and more posterior middle, superior, and supreme (when pres-

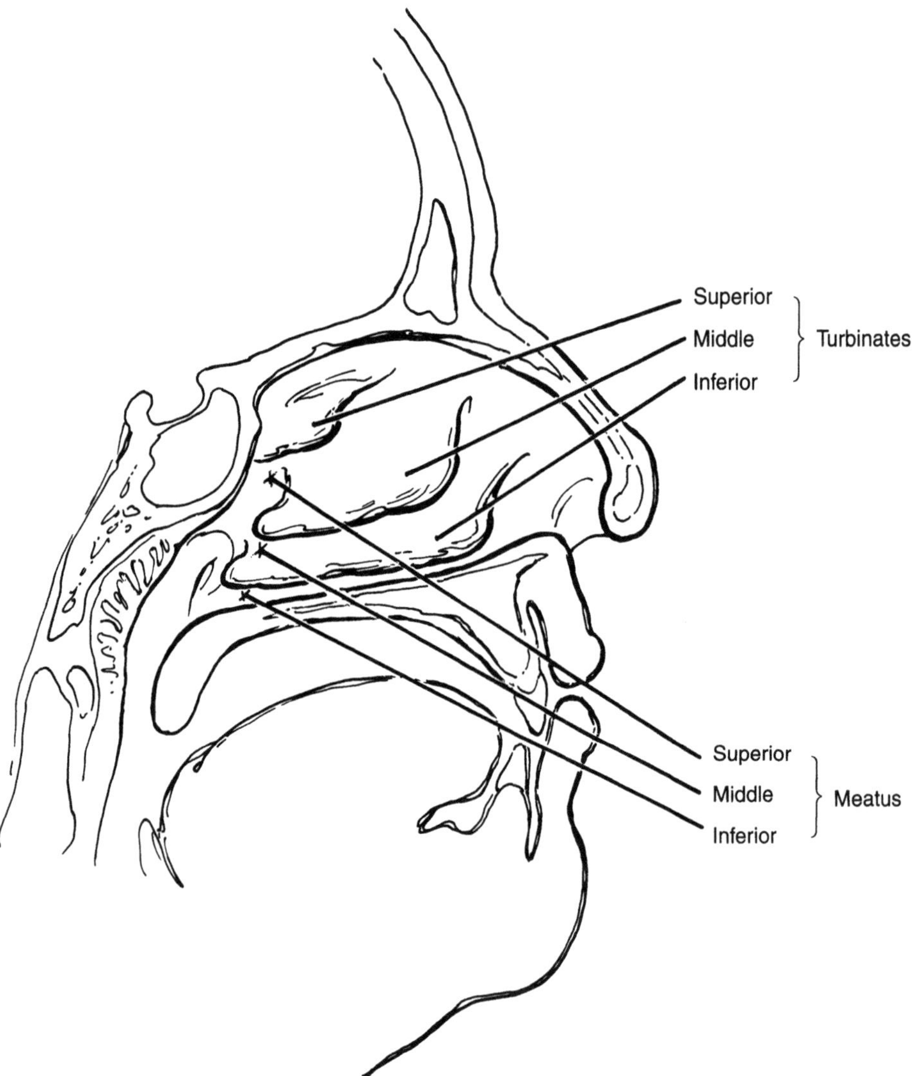

FIGURE 14.1. Nasal anatomy. Each meatal space is named for the turbinate that lies immediately above it. (Reproduced with permission from the illustrator, Virginia Cantarella, and from Lemke BN and Lucarelli MJ. Anatomy of the ocular adnexa, orbit, and related facial structures. In: Nesi FA, Lisman RD, Levine MR, eds: *Smith's Ophthalmic Plastic and Reconstructive Surgery.* 2d ed. St Louis: Mosby-Year Book 1998:9.)

External Dacryocystorhinostomy

ent) turbinates are outcroppings of the ethmoid bone. The lacrimal excretory fossa is formed by the maxillary and lacrimal bones. The nasolacrimal canal, which drains into the inferior meatus, is formed by the maxillary bone laterally and the lacrimal and inferior turbinate bones medially.

The origins of the middle turbinate are the maxillary sinus and the cribiform plate. The lacrimal sac fossa lies anterior and lateral to the anterior tip of the middle turbinate, within the widened orbital rim medially. The excretory fossa or groove is encompassed in front by the anterior lacrimal crest of the maxillary bone and behind by the posterior lacrimal crest of the lacrimal bone (Fig. 14.2). The fossa is approximately 16 mm high, 4 to 8 mm wide, and 2 mm deep,[1] and is narrower in women.[2]

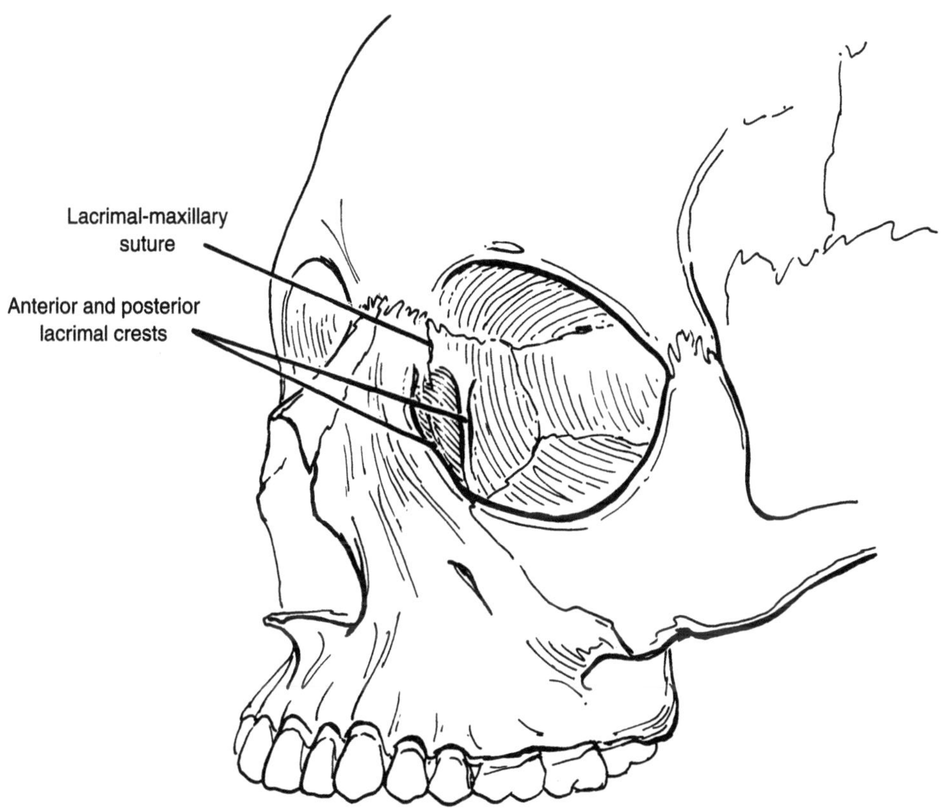

FIGURE 14.2. Lacrimal excretory fossa. (Reproduced with permission from Lemke BN and Lucarelli MJ. Anatomy of the ocular adnexa, orbit, and related facial structures. In: Nesi FA, Lisman RD, Levine MR, eds: *Smith's Ophthalmic Plastic and Reconstructive Surgery*. 2d ed. St Louis: Mosby-Year Book; 1998:14.

The anterior lacrimal crest continues as the superomedial extension of the inferior orbital rim. The anterior lacrimal crest is an important landmark during an external DCR and demarcates the anterior border of the lacrimal sac fossa. The anterior limb of the medial canthal ligament attaches to the anterior lacrimal crest superiorly. This attachment of the medial canthal ligament is often detached from the underlying bone along with the periosteum to gain better exposure during an external DCR.

A vertical suture generally runs centrally between the lacrimal and maxillary bones of the anterior and posterior lacrimal crests. The maxillary–lacrimal union may be more posteriorly placed, indicating predominance of the maxillary bone, or more anteriorly placed, indicating predominance of the lacrimal bone. In a patient with a maxillary bone–dominant fossa, the osteotomy is more difficult because of thicker bone.

Anterior ethmoidal cells termed ager nasi bullae, which rarely may also extend into the maxillary frontal process, pneumatize the lacrimal bone. Whitnall[3] found that in 54% of skulls the air cells extended anteriorly to the anterior lacrimal crest and as far as the maxillary–lacrimal suture in an additional 32%. Similarly, Blaylock et al.[4] evaluated computed tomographic (CT) scans of 190 orbits with normal ethmoid anatomy to define the anatomical relationship of anterior ethmoid air cells to the lacrimal sac fossa. In 93% of the orbits, the cells extended anterior to the posterior lacrimal crest, with 40% entering the frontal process of the maxilla. If such anatomy is not understood, a DCR fistula may be inadvertently created into the ethmoid sinus space rather than into the nasal cavity.

EVALUATION

In patients with nasolacrimal outflow obstruction, tearing is by far the most common presenting complaint. Excessive tearing can lead to severe functional impairment and visual disability, especially with reading and driving.

The preoperative evaluation of the patient with epiphora begins with a directed history, followed by an examination to determine whether the cause of the disorder is obstructive or nonobstructive. If the tearing is thought to be obstructive, it is also important to determine the site of the obstruction, since this will affect surgical management. The most common site of obstruction in both congenital and acquired lacrimal drainage disorders is the nasolacrimal duct, but obstruction can occur in any portion of the nasolacrimal drainage system, including the puncta, which can be atretic or stenotic.

Nonobstructive causes of epiphora or excess tearing include eyelid malposition (particularly entropion, ectropion, and retraction) and other ocular surface diseases predisposing the eye to irritation and reflex tearing. Conjunctivitis, conjunctivochalasis, blepharitis, and keratopathy should be excluded as potential causes of tearing. Other nonobstructive causes include thyroid ophthalmopathy, seventh cranial nerve palsy, or infrequent blinking secondary to Parkinson's disease.

Pain, redness, and swelling over the lacrimal sac are the hallmarks of acute dacryocystitis, which may cause tearing with or without mucopurulent discharge from the eye. The swelling associated with acute dacryocystitis generally is located inferior to the medial canthal tendon. Acute dacryocystitis is treated with oral and topical antibiotics as well as warm compresses. Rarely, there is a need for incision and drainage. Once the acute infection has resolved, an external dacryocystorhinostomy may be performed. Chronic dacryocystitis often leads to scarring of the nasolacrimal sac.

Nasolacrimal irrigation and probing are essential in the evaluation of patients with epiphora. To perform nasolacrimal irrigation, the authors use a 3 mL syringe with a blunt cannula needle and topical anesthetic. The medial canthal area is observed closely as water is irrigated into one of the canaliculi. Reflux of the irrigation solution via the other punctum suggests obstruction of the common canaliculus or beyond. Mucoid reflux indicates an obstruction below the lacrimal sac. Probing with a 00 Bowman probe is performed to verify the integrity of the canaliculi and the common canaliculus.

The 5-minute dye disappearance test, canaliculus irrigation test, and Jones I and Jones II tests are sometimes useful in assessing lacrimal function. In the 5-minute dye disappearance test, the ocular surface is inspected 5 minutes after instillation of fluorescein dye to determine whether there has been delay of dye passage off the ocular surface and into the nose. Patients with significant obstruction generally demonstrate substantial retention of the fluorescein on the ocular surface. As a simple procedure, the dye disappearance test is especially useful in young children.

Dacryocystography (DCG), which involves irrigation of the lacrimal drainage system with contrast material and imaging with serial radiography, is useful in studying the internal anatomy of the lacrimal system after irrigation demonstrates obstruction. Some surgeons favor DCG when a tumor of the lacrimal drainage system is suspected. In dacryoscintigraphy, a drop of technetium-99m is instilled in each conjunctival sac. As the radioisotope flows through the lacrimal drainage system mixed with tears, imaging is done with a gamma camera and mean transit times are calculated. Rates and images can be compared with those of the contralateral system and with tables of normal values. Because it does not disturb the nasolacrimal drainage system, lacrimal scintigraphy may be useful in deciding whether the patient has a lacrimal pump dysfunction or obstruction elsewhere in the system.[5,6]

Computed tomography provides excellent bony detail and is the authors' first choice for the evaluation of the tearing patient with a suspected lacrimal neoplasm or with a history of midfacial trauma. The CT scan is faster and is less expensive than a normal or high-resolution magnetic resonance imaging (MRI) scan and provides better definition of bone. Rubin et al.[7] have used high-resolution surface coil MRI effectively in selected patients with neoplastic, inflammatory, and obstructive disorders that involved the nasolacrimal system.

Nasal endoscopy can be very helpful in lacrimal evaluation, particularly in cases of failed dacryocystorhinostomies. Endoscopy should be postponed in the evaluation of the tearing patient until all other tests have been completed because nasal stimulation causes significant reflex tearing. The patient is premedicated with 20% benzocaine nasal spray (Hurricaine nasal spray, Beutlich LP Pharmaceuticals, Waukegan, IL) with or without oxymetazoline hydrochloride 0.05% nasal spray (for mucosal decongestion). It is also possible to perform endoscopy without premedication with a gentle technique, using a small (2.7 mm) endoscope.

It is important for the patient to have a thorough preoperative general medical evaluation prior to DCR surgery. A stimulant decongestant such as cocaine or epinephrine might be contraindicated in the patient with coronary arterial disease or ischemic heart disease. Medications that may lead to increased bleeding such as aspirin, nonsteroidal anti-inflammatory agents, and warfarin (Coumadin) should be discontinued prior to surgery for a period approved by the patient's primary care physician. If possible, aspirin or aspirin-containing products should be discontinued 2 weeks prior to surgery, and Coumadin should be discontinued 4 days prior to surgery. Coumadin can be restarted immediately following surgery.

In patients who cannot completely discontinue aspirin, anti-inflammatory agents, or other anticoagulant medications, the authors may nevertheless proceed cautiously with surgery. Extra precautions to prevent excess bleeding such as the use of topical thrombin and gelatin sponges (Gelfoam, Upjohn, Kalamazoo, MI) and extensive hemostasis with the monopolar cautery unit. Patients can also be switched from either aspirin or other anti-inflammatory agents to a newer cyclooxygenase-2 (COX-2) inhibitor, such as Celebrex (Pharmacia, Peapack, NJ) that does not interfere with platelet function.

TECHNIQUE

The authors usually perform external DCRs under general anesthesia on an outpatient basis. This is done primarily for patient comfort and to avoid possible respiratory complications associated with excess bleeding in the setting of a sedated patient with a compromised airway. Other authors advocate the merits of DCR under monitored sedation. In their study of outpatient DCRs, Dresner et al.[8] performed 76 of 105 procedures (72%) under monitored sedation using local anesthesia. Advantages of local anesthesia include less postoperative nausea and vomiting, reduced recovery period, and potentially less bleeding (because inhaled anesthetics are potent vasodilators).

To optimize hemostasis, 2% lidocaine with epinephrine (1:200,000) is injected into the nasal mucosa anterior to the middle turbinate. The middle meatus is packed with ribbon gauze soaked in imidazoline derivatives, such as oxymetazoline hydrochloride 0.05% nasal spray (Afrin, Schering-Plough, Madison, NJ) for hemostasis. Both these agents have hemostatic effects similar to that of cocaine, with fewer adverse cardiovascular reactions and fewer logistical problems.

When 2% lidocaine with 1:200,000 epinephrine is injected, a nasal speculum is placed in the nostril for increased visualization. The needle tip is placed into the area anterior to the middle turbinate and, after withdrawing of air to avoid injection into a vascular plexus, approximately 2 mL of the solution is injected into the nasal mucosa for hemostasis.

A surgical marker is used to outline a curvilinear incision extending from just above the level of the medial canthal tendon into the thin eyelid skin. The incision should be located lateral to the thicker skin of the nose to minimize consequent scarring. The length of the incision is approximately 15 to 20 mm and should begin at the level of the medial canthal tendon. The area surrounding the marking is then infiltrated with approximately 2 to 3 mL of 2% lidocaine with 1:200,000 epinephrine.

The skin incision is made with either a #15 Bard–Parker blade or the Colorado microdissection needle (Colorado Biomedical, Inc., Evergreen, CO) on the monopolar cautery unit. The subcutaneous and muscular dissection is carried down to the periosteum at the anterior lacrimal crest with either straight iris scissors or the cutting mode of the monopolar unit. The periosteum is incised by using the Colorado needle, and the anterior limb of the medial canthal tendon is severed. The authors attempt to avoid damage to and subsequent bleeding from the angular vessels through adequate visualization. A self-retaining retractor, Blair rake, or 4-0 silk retraction suture is used to maintain visualization of the deep tissue. Two Freer elevators are used in a hand-over-hand fashion to elevate the periosteum in all four directions and also to elevate the lacrimal sac from its fossa.

A curved hemostat or the blunt end of the Freer elevator is used to penetrate the thin lacrimal bone at the posterior aspect of the lacrimal sac fossa. If the lacrimal bone is too thick to penetrate with a hemostat or Freer elevator, the instrument can be repositioned slightly posteriorly to start the osteotomy in the thinner ethmoid bone. It is helpful at this point to remove the nasal packing to allow the nasal mucosa to move away in the event that it is contacted during bone opening. A Citelli rongeur followed by a Kerrison rongeur is then used to create a large osteotomy measuring approximately 15 × 15 mm^2.

It is very important to create a large osteotomy to increase the chance for success of the DCR. As much as one-third of the lacrimal sac fundus may lie above the medial canthal tendon. Therefore, to create an adequate osteotomy for apposition of the entire lacrimal sac and nasal mucosa, the osteotomy should extend superior to the level of the medial canthal tendon. The authors remove bone with the rongeur until thickening of the frontal bone is noted. This point should lie several millimeters above the common internal punctum.

Slightly above the level of the medial canthal tendon lies the anterior cranial fossa. Botek and Goldberg[9] found that the oblique distance between the common internal punctum and the most anterior aspect of the cribiform plate was 25.1 ± 2.95 mm, suggesting that traction or torsional forces applied to the superior bony ridge of the osteotomy could be responsible for a leak of cerebrospinal fluid. From a retrospective study of coronal maxillofacial computed tomography scans from 40 adult patients, McCann and Lucarelli[10] found that the mean vertical dimension between the medial canthal ligament and the level of the cribriform plate was 17.1 ± 4.4 mm.

As mentioned previously, ethmoid air cells may be present medial to the lacrimal sac fossa or even anterior to the lacrimal crest. These ethmoid cells should be removed to allow a proper osteotomy. Bleeding from the ethmoid air cells can occur, but usually it diminishes once the mucosa has been removed.

After creation of the bony osteotomy, attention is directed to the lacrimal sac. A Quickert–Dryden probe attached to a silicone tube or a 00 Bowman probe is passed through the superior canaliculus into the inferior portion of the lacrimal sac. By directing the tip of the probe into the inferior lacrimal sac, damage to the common internal punctum can be avoided as the sac is incised. While tenting the lacrimal sac with the probe, either a #12 Bard–Parker blade, curved Stevens scissors, or a curved crescent blade is used to open the lacrimal sac from inferior to superior along its entire length. The incision is placed posteriorly to create a large anterior mucosal flap (Fig. 14.3). Relaxing incisions are placed in the lacrimal sac mucosal flap superiorly and inferiorly. Failure to open the entire lacrimal sac may result in lacrimal sump syndrome.

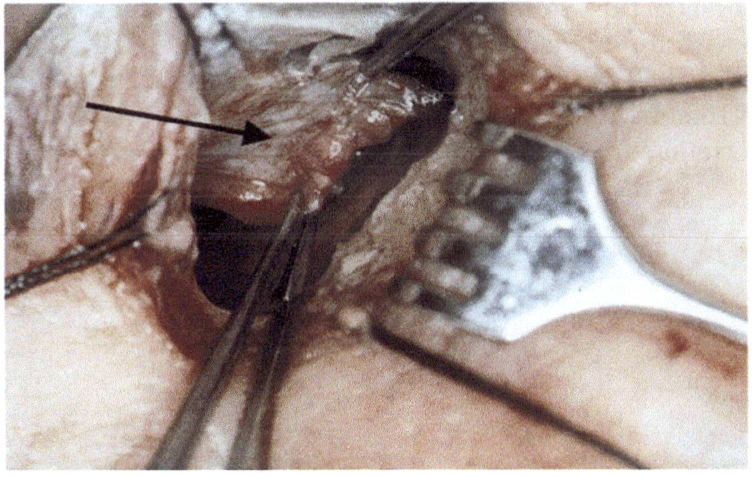

FIGURE 14.3. Lacrimal mucosal flap (arrow).

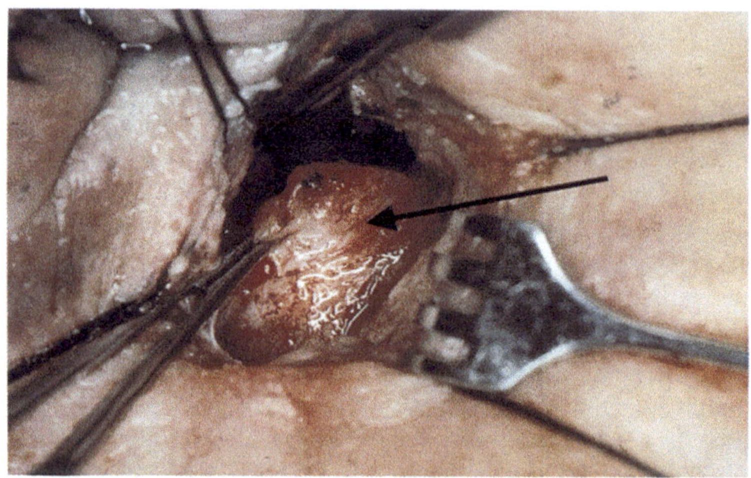

FIGURE 14.4. Nasal mucosal flap (arrow).

Attention is then directed to the nasal mucosa. Several minutes before the nasal mucosa is opened, it can be reinjected with the same lidocaine–epinephrine solution. A grooved director or Freer elevator is used to tent the nasal mucosa. Using the Colorado microdissection needle, the nasal mucosa is incised to create a large anterior-based flap (Fig. 14.4).

The silicone tubes are then passed across the ostium on the Quickert–Dryden probes. The passage of the silicone tubes through the common internal punctum and the absence of a mucosal membrane or stricture around the common internal punctum are confirmed with direct visualization. A membrane can easily lead to failure of the DCR, and any found should be excised. In an anatomical variant seen in approximately 5% of patients, the canaliculi enter the nasolacrimal sac separately.

External Dacryocystorhinostomy

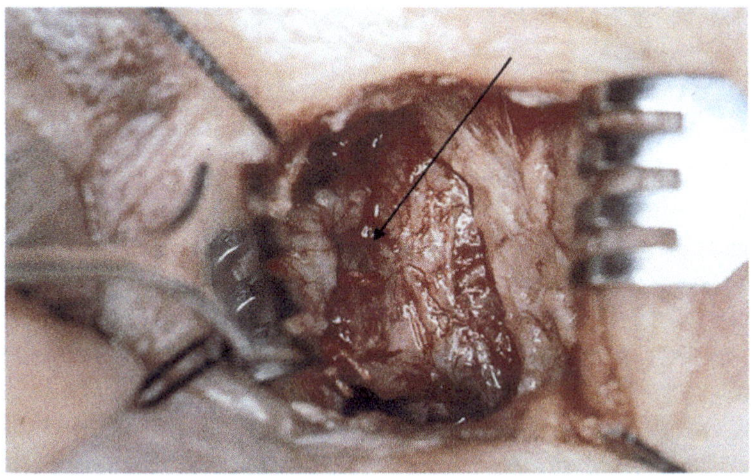

FIGURE 14.5. Approximated mucosal flaps.

The nasal mucosal flap is anastomosed to the lacrimal sac flap with interrupted 5-0 Vicryl suture (Ethicon, Somerville, NJ) (Fig. 14.5). Either flap can be trimmed to assure that there is not significant redundancy. A 5-0 Vicryl suture with a small half-circle needle (P-2) is used to close the deep orbicularis muscle, and 6-0 Vicryl suture is used to close the subcutaneous orbicularis muscle. A 6-0 fast-absorbing plain gut suture is used to reapproximate the skin edges.

The silicone tubes are gently pulled through the nose so that they assume a normal position against the eye without tension. A small hemostat is used to grasp the silicone tubes just inside the lateral vestibule. Several surgeon's knots are placed in the silicone tubes and the tubes are allowed to relax inside the nose to permit reassessment of the position of the knots against the nasal wall. A 6-0 Prolene suture is then used to secure the silicone tubes to the lateral wall of the nose.

COMPLICATIONS

Failure of the Dacryocystorhinostomy

The failure rate of an external DCR has been reported at approximately 5%.[11–14] Reasons for failure include closure or development of a membrane over the osteotomy site, formation of synechiae between the ostium and the middle turbinate or septum (Fig. 14.6), and obstruction or narrowing at the common canaliculus. Linberg et al.[15] showed that the average intraoperative bony ostium diameter was 11.84 mm, whereas the healed nasal mucosal opening measured 1.80 mm in mean diameter. In their series of 122 patients, the most common cause of failure was soft tissue obstruction of the ostium, as confirmed by office probing, nasal endoscopy, and patency of the osteotomy on CT imaging.

The authors attempt to identify common canalicular obstruction preoperatively. Similarly, during surgery, the position and condition of the common internal punctum are inspected and the superior border of the osteotomy is extended approximately 5 mm above the level of the common internal punctum. Jones[16] has recommended that a distance of at least 5 mm be created between the common internal punctum and the osteotomy margin.

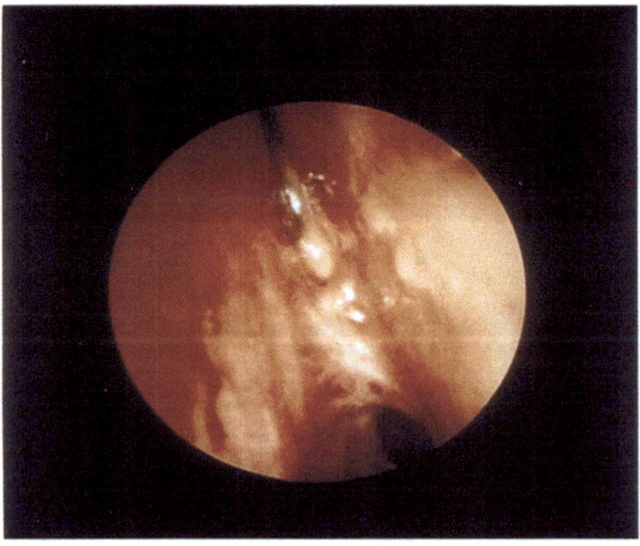

FIGURE 14.6. Formation of synechiae between the ostium and the nasal septum.

A large osteotomy is critical for maximum success with DCR surgery. Ezra et al.[17] used B-mode ultrasonography and found that the soft tissue anastomosis within the osteotomy site decreased to 49% of the immediate postoperative value by 6 months. A small osteotomy is at increased risk for soft tissue overgrowth and failure.

In the patient with a failed DCR from overgrowth of the ostium, the authors typically use the Ellman radiosurgery unit to revise the DCR endoscopically. After the soft tissue covering the osteotomy site has been confirmed, the radiosurgery unit is used to remove the granulation tissue. Mitomycin-C (0.3 mg/mL) is applied with cotton-tipped applicators in three to four applications, each lasting 2 minutes.

On the first postoperative visit, the authors irrigate the nasolacrimal drainage system to push through any clots or debris that may hinder the patency of the osteotomy site.

Hemorrhage

Hemorrhage during or following DCR can be substantial. Inactivation of the clotting cascade or platelet activity by medications such as Coumadin or aspirin is one of the main reasons for excessive intraoperative bleeding. Certain preoperative measures can minimize bleeding and decrease the chance of hemorrhage. Packing the nose with Afrin-soaked nasal gauze and injecting local anesthetic with epinephrine have been discussed previously.

Avoidance of the angular vessels is important in minimizing bleeding. Thrombin (5000 units: Gentrack, Middleton, WI) and Gelfoam help to reduce diffuse bleeding and oozing. Focal sites of bleeding are stopped with the cautery mode of the monopolar unit.

Only when there is still significant bleeding from the nose at the end of the DCR is postoperative nasal packing used. A half-inch nasal packing is covered with Bactroban antibiotic ointment (Mupirocin calcium, SmithKline Beecham, Philadelphia) and placed in the area of the middle meatus with bayonet forceps. As the packing material reaches the area of the osteotomy, the amount of bleeding usually declines dramatically. After the packing has been placed in the nose, a Freer elevator is used to compress the packing material in a superolateral direction. The packing material is removed after 3 to 4 days.

Cold compresses or ice packs are used over the DCR site continuously for the first 2 days after surgery. Heavy lifting, straining, and strenuous activity are avoided, and the patients are asked not to blow their noses for 1 to 2 weeks. Additionally, hot beverages are avoided for the first few days after surgery.

Incisional Scarring

The initial incision should be placed in the thin skin medial to the medial commissure, at the junction of the eyelid and nasal skin. Scarring is reduced if the incision is extended in a curvilinear fashion into the thin skin beneath the lower eyelid. The skin incision is not made along the side of the nose because this skin is thicker and more prone to contraction and scarring. Harris et al.[18] advocate using one of the relaxed skin tension lines in the lower eyelid for good results. With proper incision placement, careful layered closure, and postoperative ointment, scarring is rarely significant.

If a hypertrophic scar develops, the surgeon can use intensive massage, intrascar steroid injection with triamcinolone (0.25–0.50 mL, 40 mg/mL), or application of silicone sheeting (ReJuvness, ReJuvness Pharmaceuticals, Ballston Spa, NY). If the scar persists, or if an epicanthal fold develops, direct excision of the scar or multiple Z-plasties to lengthen the skin vertically may be used.

Wound Infection

Wound infection may occur following DCR, particularly in the setting of chronic or acute dacryocystitis (Fig. 14.7). The authors generally reserve intraoperative intravenous antibiotics for patients at increased risk for wound infection (including diabetics and patients with dacryocystitis). Vardy and Rose[19] have found that compared with in-

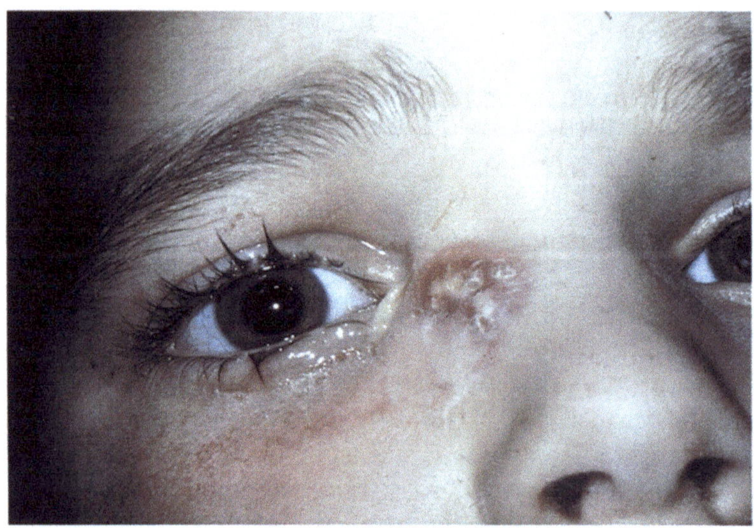

FIGURE 14.7. Right lacrimal sac infection after DCR.

External Dacryocystorhinostomy

traoperative saline lavage, intraoperative or postoperative broad-spectrum antibiotics have comparable, increased efficacy in the prevention of postoperative soft tissue cellulitis after open lacrimal surgery. They also noted that intraoperative administration of antibiotics has the advantages of compliance and lower cost. Overall, however, wound infection following DCR is uncommon.

Problems with Silicone Stents

The authors prefer to use silicone stents in all DCR surgery. In patients with canalicular or common canalicular stenosis, the stents are left in place for 6 to 9 months. If no canalicular pathology is present, removal occurs at 2 to 4 months.

The most common problem associated with silicone stents is prolapse (Fig. 14.8). Patients may dislodge the tube by rubbing the eye. Securing the tubes inside the nose may minimize this complication. Patients are also instructed about the presence and location of the silicone tube in the nose. This information is important, because patients may erroneously believe they have found an inadvertently retained "suture" in the nose. If the tubes are inadvertently pulled out, the authors attempt to reposition them by gently pushing the tube with smooth forceps back into the canaliculus. If the knotted ends of the tube are visible inside the nose, they can be resutured to the nasal wall under local anesthesia. If the tubes are entirely prolapsed, the tubes can be cut and the knotted end rotated out through one of the canaliculi.

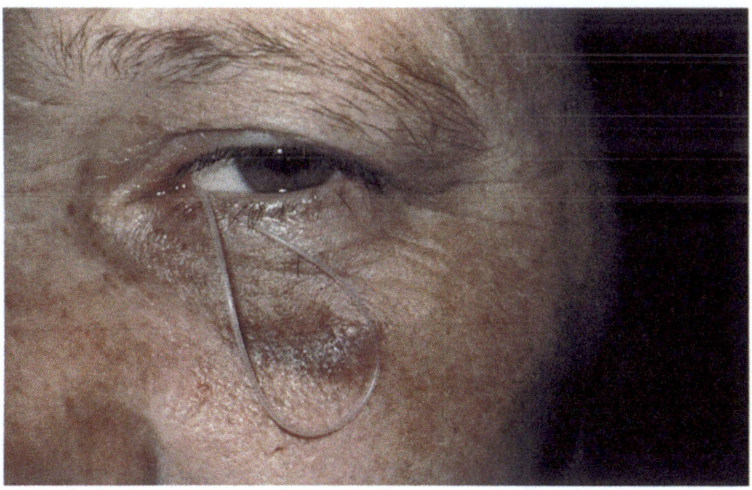

FIGURE 14.8. Prolapse of silicone lacrimal stent after DCR.

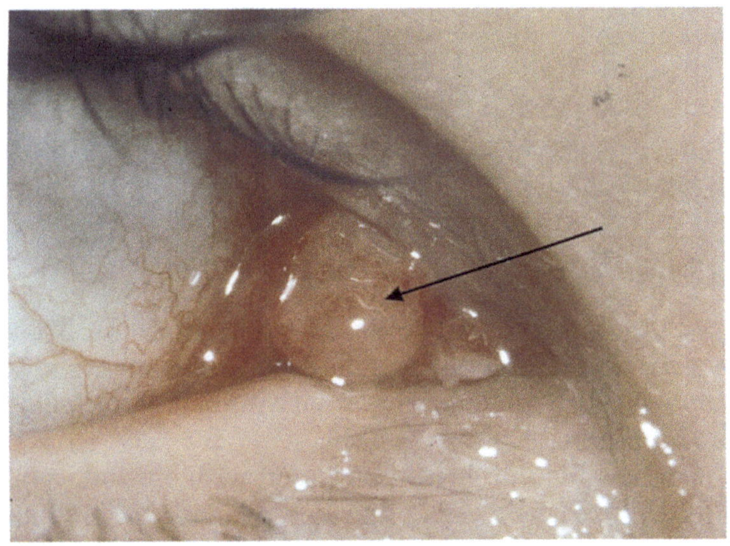

FIGURE 14.9. Granuloma around silicone tubing in right eye (arrow).

Other problems associated with silicone stents include punctal erosion and slitting of the canaliculi, formation of granulomas around the tubing (Fig. 14.9), and, rarely, corneal ulcers from abrasion by the silicone tubing (Fig. 14.10). Stent removal resolves the problem in most cases, although excision of the granuloma may be required.

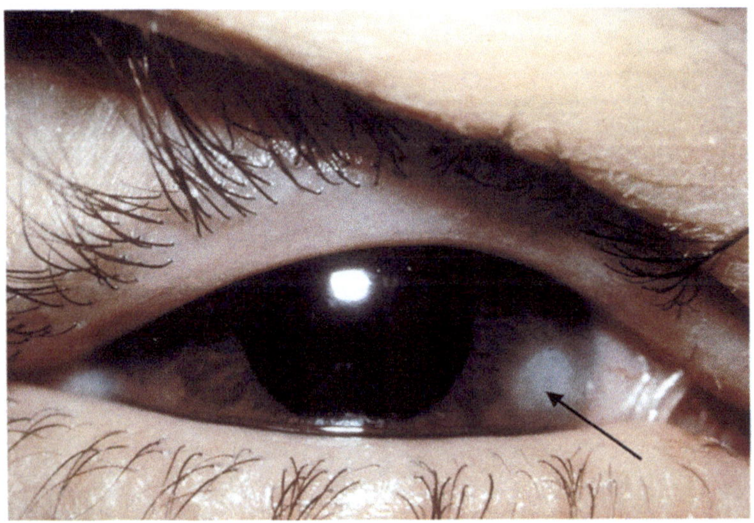

FIGURE 14.10. Corneal ulcer in right eye from abrasion by silicone tubing (arrow).

External Dacryocystorhinostomy

Cerebrospinal Fluid Leak

Cerebrospinal fluid (CSF) leak, although very uncommon, is one of the most serious complications in DCR surgery. A thorough knowledge of the anatomy of the lacrimal and ethmoidal regions can help to avoid this complication.

The medial commissure and the medial canthal tendon are landmarks during the DCR procedure. The initial skin incision is made only slightly more superior than the medial commissure and the medial canthal tendon. The osteotomy is extended the full vertical length of the lacrimal sac fossa. McCann and Lucarelli[10] found that the mean vertical dimension between the medial canthal tendon and the level of the cribiform plate was 17.1 mm ± 4.4 mm. Botek and Goldberg[9] found that the oblique distance between the common internal punctum and the most anterior aspect of the cribiform plate was 25.1 ± 2.95 mm, suggesting that traction or torsional forces applied to the superior bony ridge of the osteotomy may be responsible for a CSF leak.

If a CSF leak does occur, the surgeon should seek neurosurgical consultation if available. The site of the CSF leak will usually not be accessible through the DCR incision. Fortunately, most leaks can be managed conservatively and will close spontaneously.

ACKNOWLEDGMENTS

The authors appreciate the help of Richard K. Dortzbach, M.D., for use of his clinical and surgical photos.

REFERENCES

1. Bailey JH. Surgical anatomy of the lacrimal sac. *Am J Ophthalmol* 1923;6:665–671.

2. Lemke BN, Lucarelli MJ: Anatomy of the ocular adnexa, orbit, and related facial structures. In: Nesi FA, Lisman RD, Levine MR, eds. *Smith's Ophthalmic Plastic and Reconstructive Surgery*. 2nd ed. St. Louis: Mosby-Year Book; 1998:3–80.

3. Whitnall SE. The relations of the lacrimal fossa to the ethmoidal cells. *Ophthalmol Rev* 1911;30:321–325.

4. Blaylock WK, Moore CA, Linberg JV. Anterior ethmoid anatomy facilitates dacryocystorhinostomy. *Arch Ophthalmol* 1990;108:1774–1777.

5. Hilditch TE, Kwok CS, Amanat LA. Lacrimal scintigraphy. I. Compartmental analysis of data. *Br J Ophthalmol* 1983;67:713–719.

6. Amanat LA, Hilditch TE, Kwok CS. Lacrimal scintigraphy. II. Its role in the diagnosis of epiphora. *Br J Ophthalmol* 1983;67:720–727.

7. Rubin PAD, Bilyk JR, Shore JW, et al. Magnetic resonance imaging of the lacrimal drainage system. *Ophthalmology* 1994;101:235–243.

8. Dresner SC, Klussman KG, Meyer DR, et al. Outpatient dacryocystorhinostomy. *Ophthalmic Surg* 1991;22(4):222–224.

9. Botek AA, Goldberg RA. Margins of safety in dacryocystorhinostomy. *Ophthalmic Surg* 1993;24:320–322.

10. McCann DP, Lucarelli MJ. Radiologic analysis of the ethmoid bone–cribiform plate spatial relationship. *Invest Ophthalmol Vis Sci* 1998;39(4):abstract 2281;S498.

11. McLachlan DL, Shannon GM, Flanagan JC. Results of dacryocystorhinostomy: analysis of the reoperations. *Ophthalmic Surg* 1980;11:427–430.

12. Iliff CE. A simplified dacryocystorhinostomy. *Arch Ophthalmol* 1971;85:586–591.

13. McPherson SD, Egelston D. Dacryocystorhinostomy: a review of 106 operations. *Am J Ophthalmol* 1959;47:328–331.

14. Burns JA, Cahill KV. Modified Kinosian dacryocystorhinostomy: a review of 122 cases. *Ophthalmic Surg* 1985;16:710–716.

15. Linberg JV, Anderson RL, Bumsted RM, et al. Study of intranasal ostium external dacryocystorhinostomy. *Arch Ophthalmol* 1982;100(11):1758–1762.

16. Jones LT. The cure of epiphora due to canalicular disorders, trauma, and surgical failures on the lacrimal passages. *Trans Am Acad Ophthalmol Otolaryngol* 1962;66:506–520.

17. Ezra E., Restori M, Mannor GE, et al. Ultrasonic assessment of rhinostomy size following external dacryocystorhinostomy. *Br J Ophthalmol* 1998;82:786–789.

18. Harris GJ, Sakol PJ, Beatty RL. Relaxed skin tension line incision for dacryocystorhinostomy. *Am J Ophthalmol* 1989;108:742–743.

19. Vardy SJ, Rose GE. Prevention of cellulitis after open lacrimal surgery: a prospective study of three methods. *Ophthalmology* 2000;107(2):315–317.

15

ENUCLEATION

• Kip Dolphin

Removal of a diseased eye is intended to alleviate pain and remove serious ocular pathology. Enucleation is indicated when an eye is so severely damaged by disease, infection, or trauma that it does not provide meaningful sight and also causes intractable pain. Rehabilitation of the anophthalmic socket is intended to alleviate a loss and fill a void, both real and perceived. Despite advances in operative techniques and implant material, postoperative complications continue to occur at an unacceptable rate. Several series report a complication rate from 10 to 28%.

TECHNIQUE

General anesthesia is preferable for enucleation, especially if the patient has sustained a ruptured globe. Traction sutures of 6-0 silk, placed through the tarsus at the midpoint of the upper and lower lid margins, are used to retract the lids. A 360° conjunctival peritomy is performed. The surgeon must be careful to conserve conjunctiva, which will later be closed over the implant.

Stevens tenotomy scissors are used to bluntly divide the tissue in the intramuscular areas. Jamison muscle hooks are used to isolate the rectus muscles in succession. If the muscles will be reattached to a porous implant, the surgeon must attach sutures to the muscles.

The author prefers to fix 5-0 Vicryl sutures with spatulated needles to the muscles. After the sutures have been passed through the muscle tendon in suture ligature fashion, the muscle is divided from the globe at its tendonous insertion.

In severely inflamed eyes (i.e., endophthalmitis) or in eyes that have already undergone surgery (i.e., scleral buckling), the surgeon will encounter marked scarring between the sclera, and Tenon's capsule and orbital fat. A useful instrument that facilitates clean dissection between the sclera and adherent surrounding tissue is the Greishaber blade. Once all fascial attachments have been severed, an Alice clamp is placed on the stump of the medial rectus tendon and the eye is extorted.

A curved Kelly clamp is placed behind the eye and the optic nerve is clamped. Clamping of the nerve is performed to the achieve vasospasm of the central retinal artery. The clamp is held in place for approximately 30 seconds and then removed. Curved enucleation scissors are used to sever the optic nerve. The eye is removed and sent to pathology for examination.

If it is certain that there is no intraocular tumor and the likelihood of sympathetic ophthalmia is low (i.e., no antecedent trauma), the surgeon may use the sclera of the enucleated eye to surround the porous implant. Care must be taken to remove all pigment from the lamina fusca of the inner sclera. Additionally, the author recommends soaking the sclera in gentamicin solution (20 mg/mL) for 3 minutes if endophthalmitis is present.

The preplaced 5-0 Vicryl sutures are used to attach the muscles to the scleral wrapping of the implant. It is important to ensure proper placement of the muscles on the sclera. The rate of exposure of a porous implant increases if one fails to place the muscles 3 to 5 mm from the anterior apex of the implant. Exposure of the implant is one of the more difficult complications to deal with, so proper muscle placement is essential.

A double-layer closure is also essential to avoid exposure (Fig. 15.1). Tenon's layer is closed with a nonabsorbable suture, and then the conjunctiva is closed with an absorbable suture, usually 6-0 plain gut. The author does not insert a conformer because it may place undue tension on the suture line and increase the risk of a wound dehiscence. Omitting the conformer has not resulted in contracted sockets.

A pressure patch is essential to prevent orbital hematoma in the postoperative period. The patch should be placed at the end, while the patient is still sedated, because during emergence from general

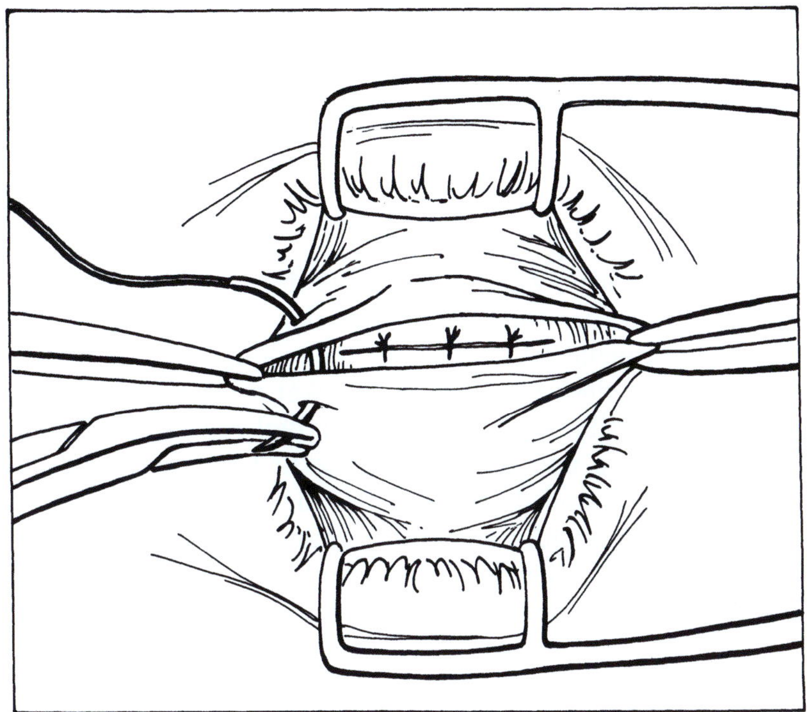

FIGURE 15.1. The double-layer closure of Tenon's capsule and conjunctiva. (Reproduced with permission, from Socket repair and reconstruction. In: Nesi FA, Gladstone GJ, Brazzo BG, et al., eds. *Ophthalmic and Facial Plastic Surgery: A Compendium of Reconstructive and Aesthetic Techniques.* Thorofare, NJ: Slack Incorporated, 2000:131.)

anesthesia the patient often struggles. The patch should remain in place for at least 4 to 5 days.

Postoperative antibiotic treatment is sometimes indicated. If endophthalmitis or panophthalmitis is present, antibiotics are necessary and should be based on culture and sensitivity. For phthisis, a 5-day course of a first-generation cephalosporin is probably adequate.

Four to 6 weeks after enucleation, the socket is generally ready for prosthesis fitting. If a porous implant drilling is planned, the surgeon must ensure that adequate vascularization has occurred. Triplephase bone scan and magnetic resonance angiography are viable methods of ensuring adequate vascularization of the implant. The practice of drilling and pegging the implant before it has become adequately vascularized leads to increased rates of infection and extrusion.

COMPLICATIONS

Complications following enucleation may involve the eyelids, implant, orbit, or socket.

Eyelids

Upper eyelid ptosis, which frequently develops after enucleation, can be corrected in the standard fashion depending on the severity of the ptosis. An external levator repair (see Chapter 6) is preferential procedure, since it does not alter the socket anatomy or shorten the superior fornix. Muller's muscle–conjunctival resection (MMCR, see Chapter 7) is a safe and predictable method for providing a small amount of elevation and does not cause significant distortion to the fornix. The surgeon should remember that direct injury to the levator or third cranial nerve may cause profound and irreversible ptosis. This situation can occur if the enucleation scissors are employed too close to the orbital apex.

Lower lid laxity is a frequent complication that becomes evident months to years after enucleation. One of the benefits of a porous implant is that it can be coupled with a peg to the prosthesis, thereby relieving the lower lid of the complete burden of supporting the prosthesis. If lower lid laxity prevents centration or retention of the prosthesis, horizontal shortening of lower lid should be undertaken (see Chapter 10). Evaluation of the attachments of the lateral and medial canthal tendons should be performed prior to surgery.

Pyogenic granuloma formation is a vexing problem for both the patient and the physician. This lesion often prevents proper fitting and placement of the prosthesis. It may produce copious mucoid discharge and bleeding. At a pathological level, pyogenic granuloma formation appears to be an aberrant attempt at tissue healing. Clinically, it may often be found in an area of wound dehiscence. Steroid drops may help to reduce the lesions. Usually, surgical excision with meticulous wound closure is necessary to treat the condition. Wound closure can be performed by direct tissue apposition, conjunctival advancement, or other more detailed steps, which will be discussed shortly in connection with exposure.

Mucoid discharge, usually due to giant papillary conjunctivitis, is a common problem. This condition arises from contact between the prosthesis and the tarsal conjunctiva. Topical agents such as steroids and mass cell stabilizers are popular treatment options. Conjunctival resection may be used in more severe cases.

The author has enjoyed good success in using 60% trichloroacetic acid topically applied to the conjunctiva with a cotton swab. Pretreatment with topical anesthetic is necessary. A dry cotton swab is dipped in the acid and applied to mucosa. The mucosa will blanch immediately. The acid is allowed to stay in contact with the tissue for as long as the patient can tolerate. When the patient signals discomfort, the socket is rinsed with copious saline. A second application may be undertaken immediately.

Implant

Implant migration is often due to muscle imbrication over the front of the implant, or a wide opening in posterior Tenon's capsule. Migration is best treated by opening the conjunctiva and repositioning the sphere in the intramuscular cone. Care should be taken not to advance the muscles too anteriorly. A double-layer closure of Tenon's and conjunctiva is advised.

The management of exposure (Fig. 15.2) and extrusion is based on the extent of the opening and the type of implant. Silastic spheres nearly always extrude once a small anterior dehiscence has occurred. If the dehiscence is small, the surgeon may try to close it with a

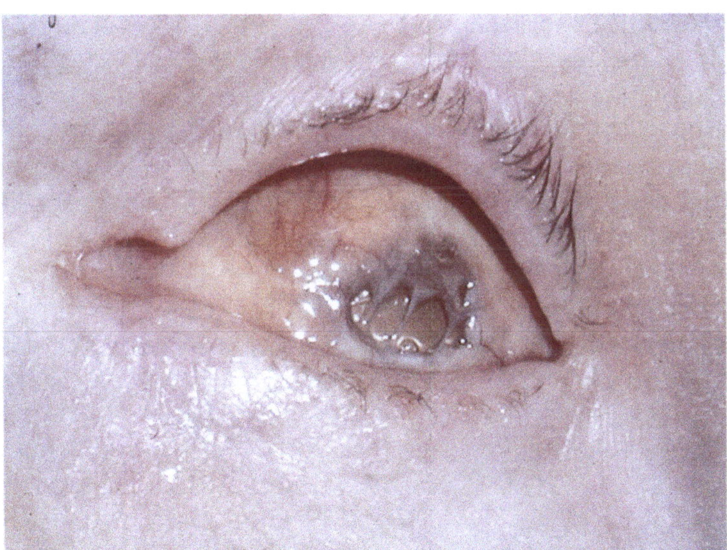

FIGURE 15.2. Conjunctival dehiscence over a silicone spherical implant.

mucosal patch graft. If the implant extrudes, the author believes that placing a dermis fat graft is the most effective option.

When exposure occurs over a porous implant, the size of the exposure dictates the course of action. If the opening is under 3 mm one may elect to observe and hope for migration and vascularization of the porous implant. During the observation period, infection of the exposed implant is a concern. If the exposure is 3 to 10 mm, repair with a buccal mucosa graft or pedicle graft of periosteum from the lateral orbital wall is a good choice. The pedicle graft has the advantage of an immediate vascular supply.

One of the advantages of porous implants is that they demonstrate good motility. This confers a natural appearance, particularly when the prosthesis is coupled to the mobile implant. In the immediate postoperative period, however, the movement of the implant imparts stress on the suture line and can promote a wound dehiscence. The author has had success with the preoperative use of botulinum toxin A (100 units in 5 mL distilled water) one week before grafting of an exposed implant. Injection may be given directly into the intraconal space behind the implant. This procedure paralyzes the extraocular muscles during the healing phase, thus preventing stress on the suture line. One must inform the patient that ptosis will occur during this 3-month period.

Peg extrusion occurs at a rate greater than most surgeons realize. In one series of 47 cases of drilling and pegging, 26% of the patients experienced extrusion of the peg. All the extrusions occurred in nonsleeved cases. The author recommends that a sleeve be placed prior to peg insertion.

Drilling of the implant prior to proper vascularization can lead to fulminate infection or rejection. One 23-year-old pregnant female was enucleated a year prior to drilling (Fig. 15.3). The surgeon, reasoned that since a year had elapsed, the implant must have vascularized, and proceeded with drilling without obtaining confirmation of adequate vascularization. Shortly after the drilling and pegging, the patient experienced progressive and inordinate pain. She underwent subtotal exenteration. Upon pathological examination, the specimen showed an orbital phlegmon surrounding a poorly vascularized hydroxyapatite implant.

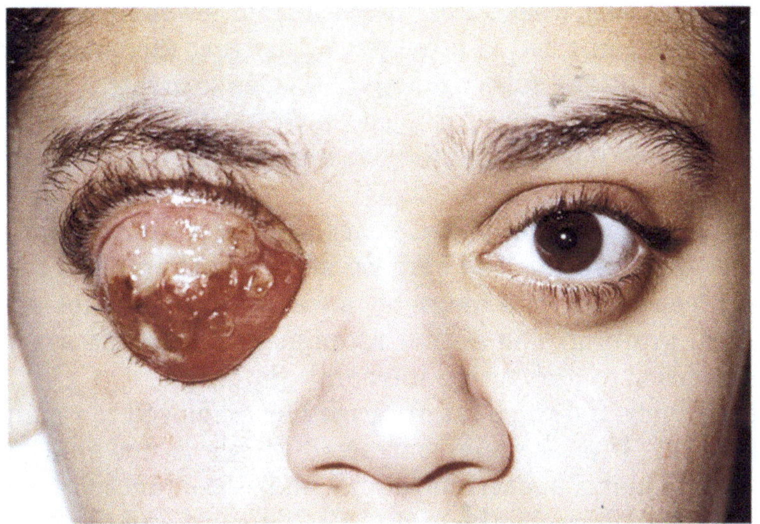

FIGURE 15.3. Formation of orbital phlegmon following drilling of orbital implant.

Orbit

Inadequate orbital volume in the anatomical socket is a common problem, which can be approached in either of two basic ways. One solution is augmentation of the intraorbital volume by placing material in the subperiosteal or intraconal space. An alloplastic material placed in the subperiosteal space gives excellent results in the author's opinion. Porous polyethylene (Medpor) is produced in different sizes for the left or right orbit and also assists in moving the spherical implant forward. A subperiosteal implant will also help to correct a deep superior sulcus. A transconjunctival approach to the inferior orbital rim allows entrance to the subperiosteal space.

Socket

Contracted socket is a formidable complication. Depending on the severity, the surgeon can either attempt to rehabilitate the socket or excise its contents and suture the lids closed. One surgical option is membrane grafting with buccal mucosa from lower lip or the lateral cheek. The recipient bed is prepared by incising the conjunctiva and bluntly dissecting the subconjunctival tissues to create a new, deeper fornix. The graft is sutured in place with 6-0 Vicryl. A conformer is placed in the new socket, and the lids are sutured together over a bolster.

Infection is a well-recognized entity, and its evaluation and prompt treatment are essential. The surgeon should keep in mind that there have been reports of actinomycetal infection of the socket after buccal mucosal grafting. The author recommends Betadine swabbing of the mouth prior to harvesting intraoral grafts.

Alternatively, a dermis fat graft may be employed to repair a contracted socket. If a severely contracted socket is not able to be repaired, the lid margins, lacrimal gland, and all conjunctiva tissue may be excised. In such cases, the orbital fat is spared and the lids are sutured closed.

16

Orbital Fractures

• Michael T. Yen
• Richard L. Anderson

The bony orbit is a component of the midfacial skeleton, and fractures often occur with facial trauma. Injuries to the eyelids, globe, sinuses, and brain can be associated with orbital fractures, and a thorough examination should be performed with particular attention to ocular and neurological function in all patients with facial trauma. Not all orbital fractures require immediate surgical intervention. The challenge for the surgeon is to recognize the clinical signs and symptoms associated with various fractures and determine which diagnostic, medical, and surgical treatments are required for each individual patient. A multidisciplinary approach with the neurosurgeon, the otolaryngologist, and the oral surgeon may be indicated for severe facial injuries.

Since the medial wall and floor are the thinnest bones of the orbit, they are easily and most commonly fractured, even from mild, seemingly insignificant trauma. Isolated fractures of the floor or medial wall without involvement of the orbital rim are classified as indirect or "blowout" fractures. One theory proposes that retropulsion of the globe hydraulically increases orbital pressure to the thin bony walls, causing them to rupture outward.[1] The globe does not rupture because this would call for a significantly higher amount of force than is needed to rupture the orbital floor or medial wall.[2] Another theory suggests that direct trauma to the inferior orbital rim transmits force posteriorly, causing a compression fracture, or buckling, of the orbital floor.[3] Both theories have scientific support, and susceptibility to a particular mechanism of injury may be related to individual anatomical variation.[2]

Lateral wall, orbital rim, and orbital roof fractures may be present in more severe injuries. Anterior impact forces cause fractures along the lines of weakness in the midfacial skeleton as described by Le Fort.[4] Often complex and asymmetric, these fractures may involve the zygoma, maxilla, nasal, and lacrimal bones. Lateral impact forces tend to be centered on the prominence of the zygoma, resulting in fractures to the zygomatic–maxillary complex. The fractures are usually located at the zygomaticofrontal suture, the zygomaticomaxillary suture, and near the midpoint of the zygomatic arch.[4] The orbital floor and maxillary sinus are often also fractured in conjunction with the zygomatic components. The orbital roof may be fractured with direct trauma to the frontal bone.[5] Although infrequent, such fractures may be seen in conjunction with frontal sinus, cribiform plate, and intracranial injury.

The bones of the orbital apex can also be fractured in association with other fractures of the face and orbit.[6] These fractures are often difficult to manage owing to the high risk of optic nerve dysfunction from compression by edema and bone, and from disruption of its vascular supply. After initial treatment with high doses of intravenous corticosteroids, bony decompression of the canal should be performed only if a bone fragment is impinging on the optic nerve or if documented compressive visual loss is progressing.

EVALUATION

Clinical

Whenever possible, a detailed history should be obtained to determine the type and extent of injuries. For example, missile injuries often perforate the orbits and result in intracranial penetration. The patient's neurological status should be given immediate attention under these circumstances. Life-threatening complications such as intracranial hemorrhage or vascular compromise of the great vessels of the neck should be treated before the orbital injuries are addressed.

A thorough examination of the periorbital region should be performed in all patients with facial trauma. The orbital rim should be palpated, with assessment for displaced fractures. The axial position of the globes should be noted with a Hertel exophthalmometer. Enophthalmos may be present in large floor or medial wall fractures. Proptosis may occur secondary to retrobulbar hemorrhage and edema. Bisecting each medial canthus with a ruler and estimating the vertical position of the pupil may permit the surgeon to detect hypophthalmos on the injured side. Binocular diplopia with limitations of extraocular movements may be seen with entrapment of orbital tissue or the extraocular muscles within the fracture (Fig. 16.1). Forced duction testing should be performed to differentiate between entrapment and paresis of the inferior rectus muscle. Hypoesthesia in the distribution of the infraorbital nerve and emphysema of the eyelids are both suggestive of orbital wall fractures.

A careful ophthalmic examination should be performed to rule out ocular injury. If possible, a baseline assessment of visual acuity should be obtained. Particular attention should be focused on the presence of penetrating injuries, intraocular hemorrhage, increased intraocular pressure, retinal detachment, and optic nerve perfusion and edema. Any ocular abnormalities should be addressed prior to intervention for the orbital injuries. Ruptured globes should be repaired prior to orbital fracture repair, since orbital manipulation may cause extrusion of intraocular contents.

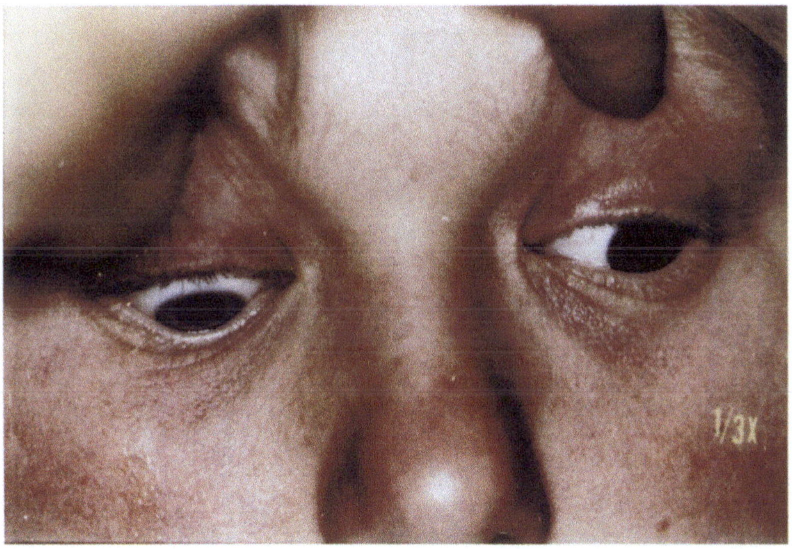

FIGURE 16.1. A 12-year-old girl with a left orbital blowout fracture 4 days after injury: 3 mm of enophthalmos is present, resulting in a smaller palpebral fissure height. Marked restriction of extraocular motility is present in downgaze.

Radiographic

Radiographic studies should be obtained for all facial injuries. Although orbital fractures can be detected with plain film radiographs such as Caldwell and Waters views, computed tomography (CT) scans are more sensitive for detecting orbital fractures.[7] Axial views can provide evidence of medial wall and zygomatic fractures. Coronal views are best for detecting orbital floor, medial wall, orbital roof, and orbital rim fractures (Fig. 16.2). Opacification of the superior maxillary sinus, just under an orbital floor fracture, may be indicative of entrapped orbital tissue within the fracture. If optic nerve injury is suspected, fine cuts (1 mm) of the optic canals should be obtained to determine the presence of optic nerve compression from bone fragments.

It has been the authors' clinical experience that CT scans underestimate the size of most orbital fractures. Some scans show little displacement of the orbital floor, yet surgical exploration reveals a large fracture with entrapment of orbital tissues. This is particularly true for young individuals with "trapdoor"-type fractures, in which a significant amount of tissue entrapment is present without radiographic

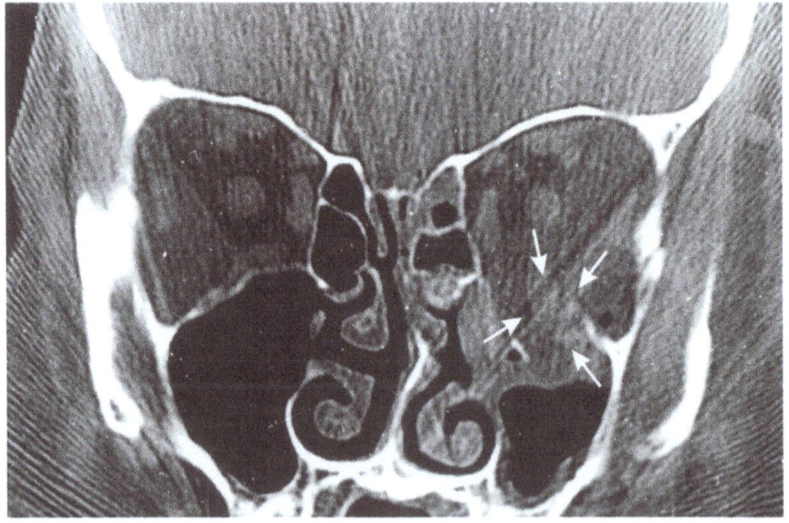

FIGURE 16.2. CT scan showing a large orbital floor fracture after assault injury to the left orbit. The inferior rectus muscle (outlined by arrows) is prolapsing through the fracture into the maxillary sinus.

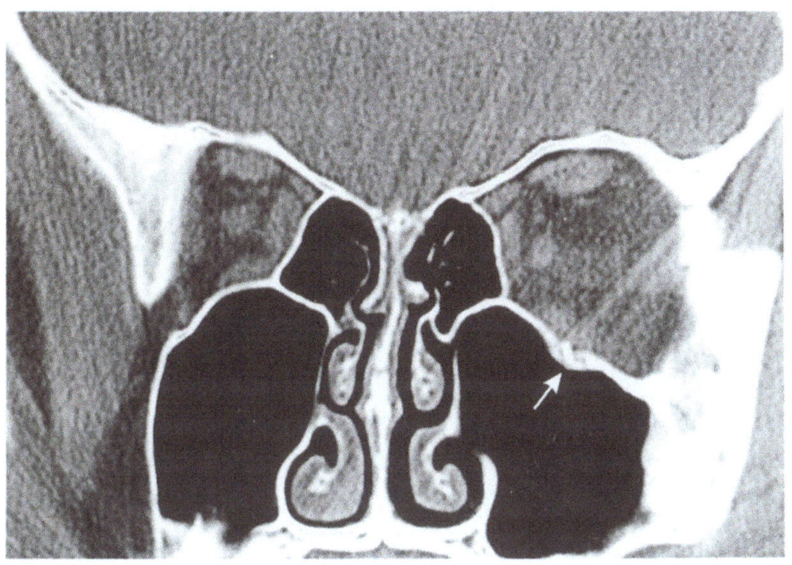

FIGURE 16.3. A 12-year-old girl with very little clinical evidence of trauma nevertheless had marked restriction of extraocular movements. This CT image shows a minimally displaced orbital floor (arrow).

evidence of a large fracture (Fig. 16.3).[8] CT scans should be used only in conjunction with the clinical examination to determine whether surgical intervention is necessary.

Surgical Indications

Many patients with orbital fractures do not require surgical repair.[9] Nondisplaced fractures or asymptomatic patients can be treated with observation alone. Displaced orbital rim and zygomatic fractures require open reduction and internal fixation. Without surgical intervention, the patient may develop flattening of the malar prominence, lateral canthal dystopia, and jaw malocclusion with pain on mastication.

For blowout fractures, the accepted indications for surgical repair include diplopia with entrapment of orbital tissues, greater than 2 mm of enophthalmos, large fractures involving more than 50% of the orbital floor, and intractable pain with extraocular movements. Since orbital edema and hemorrhage can impair extraocular motility as well as cause some degree of proptosis, the authors recommend that adults be observed for 7 to 10 days after the injury, to allow resolution of the edema and hemorrhage. If surgical indications remain after this period of observation, repair should be performed within 2 to 3 weeks of the injury, prior to the development of significant scar tissue formation.

There is growing evidence that children with orbital fractures should undergo early surgical repair, within days of the injury.[8,10,11] Early intervention is desirable to prevent the development of inferior rectus muscle fibrosis as well as to provide more rapid improvement in motility. The bones in children are also more pliable, and "trapdoor"-type fractures are common. For children, the authors recommend early surgical repair for all orbital fractures that appear to be clinically entrapped. Postoperative fibrosis of the inferior rectus muscle may still develop despite early surgical intervention, and these children should be followed closely with the assistance of a pediatric ophthalmologist.

TECHNIQUES

Repair of Blowout Fractures

Since repair of orbital fractures often involves posterior orbital exploration, general anesthesia is usually required. The authors prefer to access the orbit through a transconjunctival lower eyelid incision to minimize the risk of eyelid retraction and prominent scarring.[12] In conjunction with a lateral canthotomy and cantholysis, excellent exposure of the medial wall, orbital floor, and majority of the lateral wall can be obtained with the transconjunctival approach. Other methods for entering the orbit include a subciliary, transbuccal transantral (Caldwell–Luc), or coronal approach.

Local anesthetic (2% lidocaine with epinephrine) is infiltrated into the inferior fornix as well as the lateral canthal region. Forced duction testing is first performed to obtain a baseline assessment of ocular motility. With forceps, the surgeon grasps the insertion of the inferior rectus muscle through the conjunctiva and attempts to move the globe superiorly and inferiorly. The same maneuver is done with the medial rectus, attempting to move the globe horizontally.

The amount of lower eyelid laxity is then assessed by retracting inferiorly with a Desmarres retractor. If the lower eyelid cannot be retracted to the inferior orbital rim, then a lateral canthotomy with inferior cantholysis as discussed in Chapter 10 (see Figs. 10.3 and 10.4) is typically required to provide adequate access to the orbital floor. Lateral orbital wall and rim fractures often require canthotomy with inferior and superior cantholysis to provide adequate exposure of the fractures.

The transconjunctival incision is created with scissors halfway between the lower tarsal border and the inferior fornix. With floor fractures, the width of the incision should be from the lateral canthus to the caruncle. With medial wall fractures, the incision may be carried anterior or posterior to the caruncle, then superiorly to provide greater exposure. The conjunctiva and capsulopalpebral fascia are then separated from the anterior lamella (skin and orbicularis) and elevated superiorly with a 4-0 silk traction suture (Fig. 16.4). While the eyelid is retracted inferiorly and protected with the Desmarres retractor, dissection is performed down to the inferior orbital rim. The periosteum is then incised with a #15 Bard–Parker blade along the orbital rim. A Freer elevator is used to initiate the separation of the

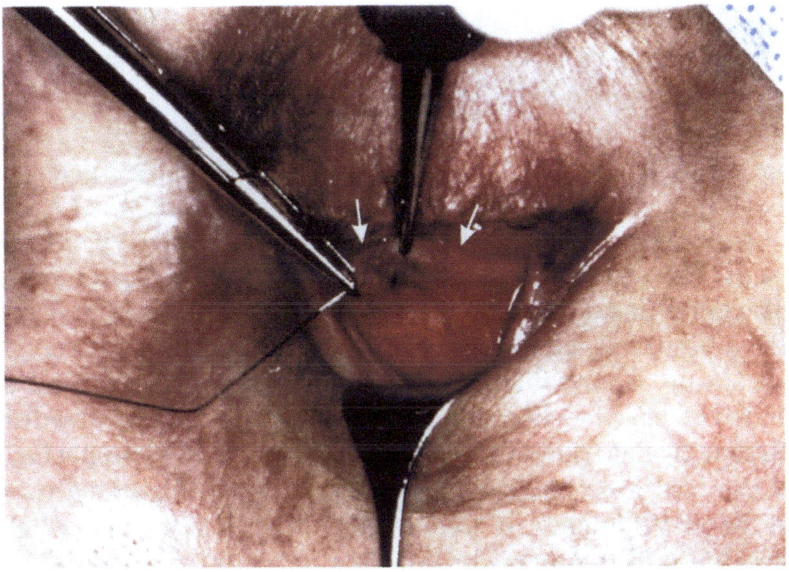

FIGURE 16.4. After the transconjunctival incision has been created from the lateral canthus to the caruncle, the conjunctiva and capsulopalpebral fascia (arrows) are separated from the anterior lamella and elevated superiorly with a traction suture.

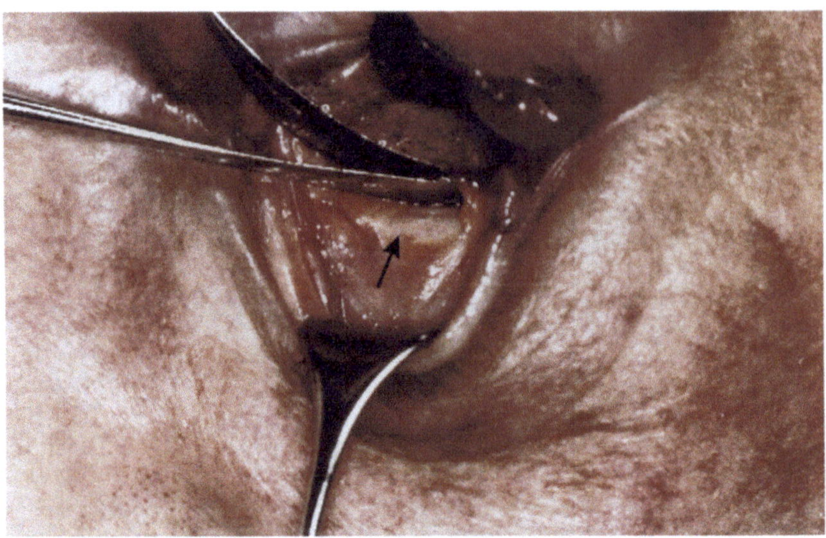

FIGURE 16.5. After the periosteum has been incised with a blade, a Freer elevator is used to initiate the separation of the periosteum from the orbital floor (arrow points to orbital rim).

periosteum from the orbital floor (Fig. 16.5). Two Sewall retractors can then be used to further elevate the periosteum superiorly and posteriorly to provide exposure of the fracture site.

Once the fracture has been located, orbital tissue will be seen herniating through the bony defect. This tissue must be gently mobilized back into the orbit. The authors prefer a "hand-over-hand" technique using the two Sewall retractors. If a trapdoor type of fracture is present, the orbital floor may need to be gently depressed to free the entrapped tissue. In older fractures, where fibrosis and scarring may have occurred, gentle traction may be required to free the entrapped tissue. Sharp dissection is usually not required and should be avoided if possible because it increases the risk of bleeding and inadvertent transection of the extraocular muscles. The posterior extent of the fracture should be identified and all entrapped tissue released. Bone fragments or depressions within the sinus should be manipulated with a muscle hook to try to reapproximate the floor or removed from the fracture site.

Once the entire fracture has been visualized, it should be completely covered with an implant. The authors' implant of choice is a sheet of porous polyethylene (Medpor, Porex Surgical, College Park,

GA). This implant material is relatively inexpensive and is easily cut to the desired shape. The porous nature of the implant allows for fibrovascular ingrowth, which minimizes implant migration and infection.[13] The Medpor sheet is cut to mold to the entire orbital floor and minimize displacement (Fig. 16.6). When properly sized, the implant will fit snugly, just posterior to the inferior orbital rim, and prevent anterior migration. If the floor fracture is particularly large with minimal stable bone along the orbital floor, a titanium microplate fixated to the orbital rim can be used to provide support for the floor implant. After the implant has been positioned, thorough exploration should

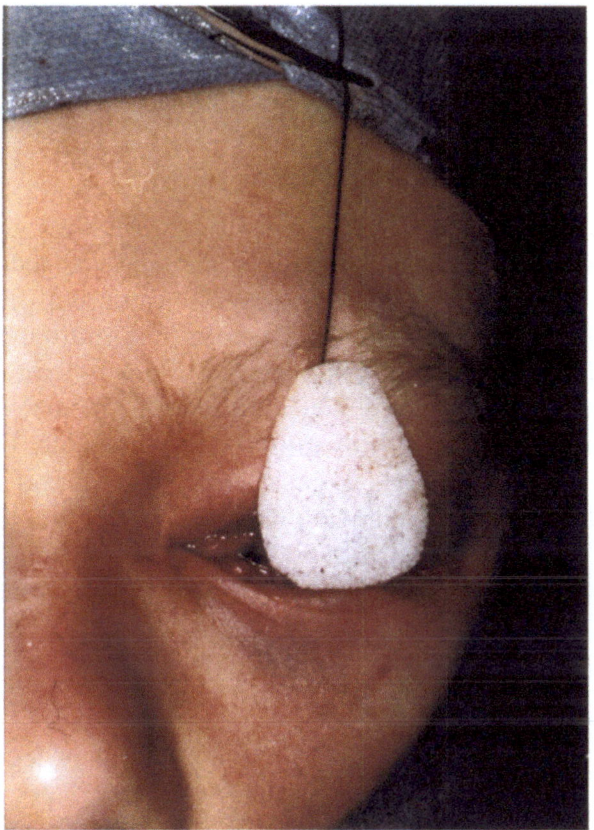

FIGURE 16.6. After all the entrapped tissue is released, a porous polyethylene implant is cut to fit the entire orbital floor and minimize displacement.

confirm that there has been no additional entrapment of orbital tissues by the implant.

Forced duction testing is repeated prior to and after placing the implant to demonstrate improvement of ocular motility and to confirm that tissue was not entrapped around the edges of the implant. The periosteum is then closed with interrupted 4-0 Vicryl sutures. The transconjunctival incision is approximated with interrupted 6-0 plain gut sutures. If a lateral canthotomy was created, the lower eyelid is secured with 4-0 Vicryl sutures to the periosteum of the lateral orbital rim or the superior crus of the lateral canthal tendon. The canthal skin is then reapproximated with an interrupted 6-0 plain gut suture, and the remainder of the canthotomy incision is closed with interrupted 6-0 plain gut sutures. If there are no contraindications, the authors prefer to place all patients undergoing repair of orbital fractures on a tapering dose of oral corticosteroids for the first postoperative week.

Repair of Displaced Orbital Rim and Zygomatic Fractures

Exposure of all fracture sites must be achieved before reduction and fixation.[14] We prefer to use a transconjunctival incision to provide exposure of the entire inferior orbital rim and superior maxilla. When combined with cantholysis, such an incision can easily expose the lateral orbital rim up to the zygomaticofrontal suture.[15] For lower maxillary fractures, a superior gingival incision may be required as well. In fractures with minimal displacement, a large bone hook or an Alice clamp may be used to elevate and rotate the bone to reduce the fracture. If more severe displacement is present, additional approaches such as a Gillies temporal approach or a gingival approach may be required to provide adequate leverage on the zygoma to elevate it into the proper position (Fig. 16.7). Accurate reduction of these fractures is important to reestablish the normal width, height, and projection of the midface.

After reduction of the fractures, rigid fixation with titanium microplates is performed. The authors prefer to use the smallest and thinnest plates available except on the zygomatic arch, where a larger plate may be required to resist the forces of the masticatory muscles. The length of the plate should extend several millimeters past the fracture to allow placement of at least two fixation screws on each side of the fracture. Rigid fixation should be placed on at least two fracture sites, most commonly the zygomaticofrontal and the zygo-

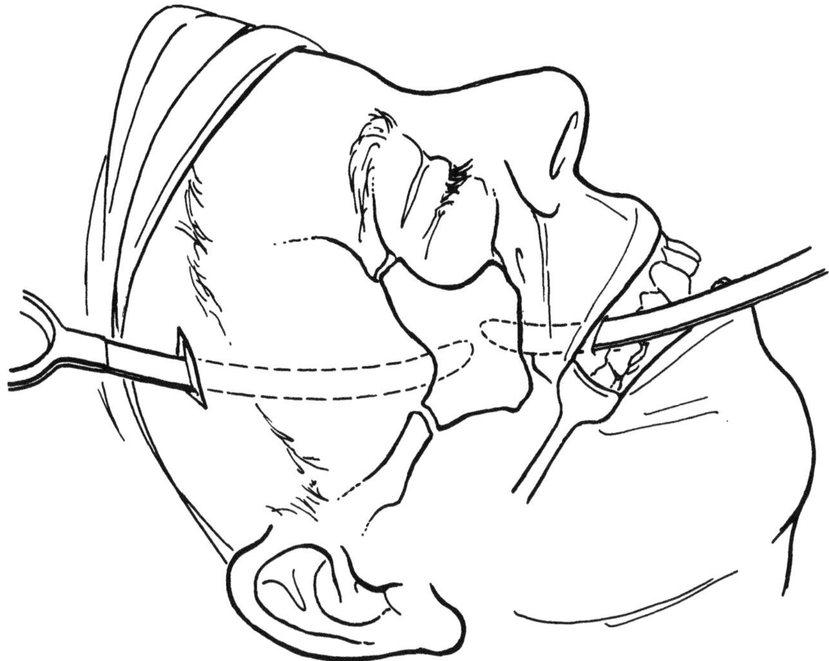

FIGURE 16.7. Fracture reduction may require a gingival or temporal incision. (Reproduced with permission from Orbital fractures. In: Nesi FA, Gladstone GJ, Brazzo BG, et al, eds. *Ophthalmic and Facial Plastic Surgery: A Compendium of Reconstructive and Aesthetic Techniques*. Thorofare, NJ: Slack Incorporated, 2000:126.)

maticomaxillary sutures, to achieve greatest stability and alignment. Inadequate reduction and fixation may lead to facial asymmetry with flattening of the malar prominence.

COMPLICATIONS

The potential complications of orbital fracture repair should be explained to all patients, regardless of the size and severity of the injuries, by means of appropriate counseling. The most serious complication is a visual loss, which may be caused by direct optic nerve injury, ciliary or retinal artery occlusion, retrobulbar hemorrhage, or compression of the optic nerve by the implant. Careful tissue manipulation, meticulous hemostasis, and proper sizing and placement of the implant can help to avoid this problem.[16]

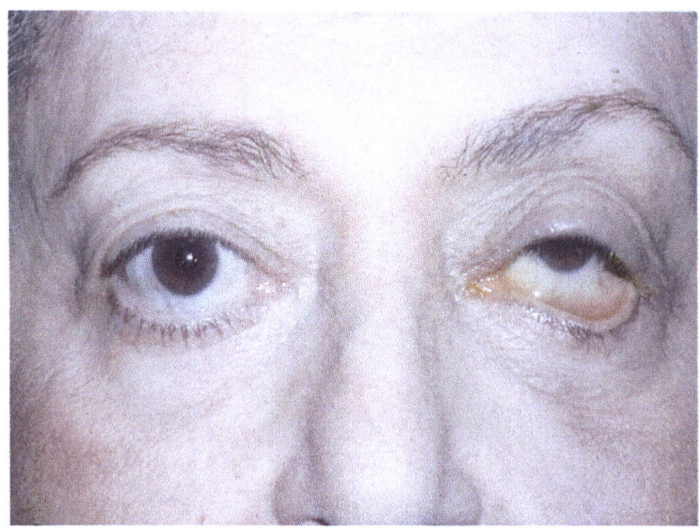

FIGURE 16.8. Following transcutaneous repair of a left inferior orbital wall fracture, scar tissue developed and caused severe ectropion and retraction. This patient also developed mild hypertropia.

If a transcutaneous approach is used to access the orbital floor, postoperative malposition of the lower eyelid (Fig. 16.8) may develop. Scarring of the orbicularis muscle to the orbital septum and periosteum leads to lower eyelid retraction. This complication can be avoided with the transconjunctival incision. Lower eyelid retraction can still develop when a transconjunctival incision is used if inappropriate closure of the periosteum incarcerates the orbital septum or the orbicularis muscle. Meticulous technique with good knowledge of eyelid anatomy is crucial to avoid this complication.[17]

Some degree of diplopia is common after repair of the orbital fracture. This effect is primarily due to postoperative orbital edema. The authors prefer to give a tapering dose of oral corticosteroids to minimize the amount of postoperative edema and hasten its resolution. Persistent or more severe diplopia after resolution of edema can be due to incomplete fracture reduction, entrapment of orbital tissues by the implant, or fibrosis and scar tissue formation. Complete visualization of the fracture margins with release of all entrapped tissues is important to minimize the risk of these complications. Before leaving the operating room after placement of the implant, the surgeon should also perform forced duction testing to ensure that no restrictive component is present. Occasionally, additional surgical exploration is required to release adhesions and fibrosis. In children, fibrosis of the inferior rectus muscle can occur, and strabismus surgery may be required later to alleviate diplopia.

Inferior rectus paresis may also contribute to postoperative diplopia. This situation may be due to the initial trauma or to prolonged entrapment, contusion, or hemorrhage. Serial examinations should be performed over several months to assess for improvement or stability. If symptomatic diplopia persists, the patient can be treated with prisms or strabismus surgery.

Persistent or late enophthalmos is not uncommon. It can be due to initial undercorrection of enophthalmos, or to late atrophy of the orbital fat.[16] When correcting blowout fractures, the authors prefer to have an acute exophthalmos of the surgical side, since orbital edema causes a few millimeters of proptosis that will resolve postoperatively. For correction of cosmetically unacceptable enophthalmos, a variety of implants are available to provide volume replacement. The authors prefer to use a porous polyethylene enophthalmos wedge, which is contoured to the shape of the orbital floor and provides more posterior volume replacement.

Implant migration is significantly decreased when porous implants are used. The porosity allows for fibrovascular tissue ingrowth, which helps to integrate and fixate the orbital implants.[13] This characteristic also reduces the risk of postoperative infections in the implant. Proper sizing of the implant can also reduce the risk of migration during the early postoperative period.

REFERENCES

1. Smith B, Regan WFJ. Blowout fracture of the orbit: mechanism and correction of inferior orbital fracture. *Am J Ophthalmol* 1957;44:73–39.

2. Warwar RE, Bullock JD, Ballal DR, Ballal RD. Mechanisms of orbital floor fractures: a clinical, experimental, and theoretical study. *Ophthalmic Plast Reconstr Surg* 2000;16:188–200.

3. Kersten RC. Blow-out fracture of the orbital floor with entrapment caused by isolated trauma to the orbital rim. *Am J Ophthalmol* 1987;103:215–219.

4. Stanley RB. Maxillary and periorbital fractures. In: Bailey BJ, ed. *Head and Neck Surgery—Otolaryngology*. Philadelphia: Lippincott, 1993:973–990.

5. McLachlan DL, Flanagan JC, Shannon GM. Complications of orbital roof fractures. *Ophthalmology* 1982;89:1274–1278.

6. Anderson RL, Panje WR, Gross CE. Optic nerve blindness following blunt forehead trauma. *Ophthalmology* 1982;89:445–455.

7. Nesi FA, Spoor TC. Orbital fractures. In: Nesi FA, Lisman RD, Levine MR, Brazzo BG, Gladstone GJ, eds. *Smiths Ophthalmic Plastic and Reconstructive Surgery*. St. Louis: Mosby-Year Book; 1998:205–208.

8. Jordan DR, Allen LH, White J, et al. Intervention within days for some orbital floor fractures: the white-eyed blowout. *Ophthalmic Plast Reconstr Surg* 1998;14:379–390.

9. Putterman AM, Stevens T, Urist MJ. Non-surgical management of blow-out fracture of the orbital floor. *Am J Ophthalmol* 1974;77:232–239.

10. Bansagi ZC, Meyer DR. Internal orbital fractures in the pediatric age group: characterization and management. *Ophthalmology* 2000;107:829–836.

11. Egbert JE, May K, Kersten RC, Kulwin DR. Pediatric orbital floor fracture: direct extraocular muscle involvement. *Ophthalmology* 2000;107:1875–1879.

12. Tenzel RR, Miller GR. Orbital blow-out fracture repair, conjunctival approach. *Am J Ophthalmol* 1971;71:1141–1142.

13. Rubin PAD, Bilyk RJ, Shore JW. Orbital reconstruction using porous polyethylene sheets. *Ophthalmology* 1994;101:1697–1708.

14. Glassman RD, Manson PN, Vanderkolk CA, et al. Rigid fixation of internal orbital fractures. *Plast Reconstr Surg* 1990;86:1103–1109.

15. Dolan RW, Smith DK. Superior cantholysis for zygomatic fracture repair. *Arch Facial Plast Surg* 2000;2:181–186.

16. Koh JY, Della Rocca R, Mayer EA. Orbital floor fractures: diagnosis and management. In: Naugle TC, ed. *Diagnosis and Management of Oculoplastic and Orbital Disorders*. New York: Kugler; 1994:271–284.

17. Kersten RC, Kulwin DR. Orbital blowout fractures. In: Tse DT, ed. *Color Atlas of Ophthalmic Surgery: Oculoplastic Surgery*. Philadelphia: Lippincott; 1992: 35–48.

INDEX

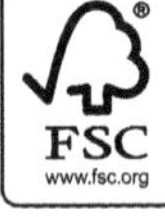